THEORY IN SCHOOL-BASED OCCUPATIONAL THERAPY PRACTICE

A Practical Application

THEORY IN SCHOOL-BASED OCCUPATIONAL THERAPY PRACTICE

A Practical Application

Patricia Laverdure, OTD, OTR/L, BCP, FAOTA

Old Dominion University
Norfolk, Virginia

Francine M. Seruya, PhD, OTR/L, FAOTA

Mercy College
Dobbs Ferry, New York

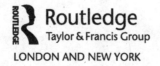

Routledge
Taylor & Francis Group

LONDON AND NEW YORK

Designed cover image: Tinhouse Design

First published 2024
by Routledge
605 Third Avenue, New York, NY 10158

and by Routledge
4 Park Square, Milton Park, Abingdon, Oxon, OX14 4RN

Routledge is an imprint of the Taylor & Francis Group, an informa business

© 2024 Taylor & Francis

ISBN: 9781630917715 (pbk)
ISBN: 9781003526773 (ebk)

DOI: 10.4324/9781003526773

Typeset in Minion Pro
by SLACK Incorporated

CONTENTS

ABOUT THE AUTHORS

Patricia Laverdure, OTD, OTR/L, BCP, FAOTA, is an associate professor and founding program director of the doctor of occupational therapy program at Old Dominion University and Eastern Virginia Medical School in Norfolk, Virginia. She has worked with children and youth and their families across the care continuum from neonatal intensive care and inpatient and outpatient services to early intervention and school services in roles of provider, consultant, and program administrator.

Dr. Laverdure codeveloped the quality indicators for school-based practice to advance professional reasoning, innovation, and learning; participation; and health/wellness outcomes in educational practice. She served as the American Occupational Therapy Association Early Intervention and Schools Special Interest Section chair and currently serves as the American Occupational Therapy Association Special Interest Section council chair.

Francine M. Seruya, PhD, OTR/L, FAOTA, is a professor and program director of occupational therapy at Mercy College in Dobbs Ferry, New York. She has been a pediatric occupational therapist for more than 2 decades working with children and their families in a variety of settings, including early intervention, preschool, and K–12 settings.

Dr. Seruya has served as the editor of the American Occupational Therapy Association Early Intervention and Schools and the Academic Education Special Interest section. She has authored numerous publications related to the use of coaching models in pediatric practice, the exploration of professional identity in school-based practice, and the phenomenon of collaboration in school-based settings.

CONTRIBUTING AUTHORS

Tammy Blake, OTD, OTR/L (Chapter 7)
Pediatric Occupational Therapist
Physical and Occupational Therapy Services
Fairfax County Public Schools
Fairfax, Virginia

Mindy Garfinkel, OTD, OTR/L, ATP (Chapter 9)
Program Director
Occupational Therapy Doctorate Program
Yeshiva University
Bronx, New York

Moses N. Ikiugu, PhD, OTR/L, FAOTA
Professor and Director of Research
Occupational Therapy Department
University of South Dakota
Vermillion, South Dakota

Paula Kramer, PhD, OTR, FAOTA
Professor Emeritus
University of the Sciences
Philadelphia, Pennsylvania

Deborah Schwind, DHSc, OTR/L, BCP, SCSS, FAOTA (Chapter 6)
Pediatric Occupational Therapist
Ashburn, Virginia

Caitlin Stanford, OTD, OTR/L (Chapter 8)
Occupational Therapist
Montville Township Public Schools
Montville, New Jersey

Miranda Virone, OTD, OTR/L (Chapter 11)
Assistant Professor of Occupational Therapy
Slippery Rock University
Slippery Rock, Pennsylvania

Tina Weisman, OTD, OTR/L (Chapter 10)
Adjunct Professor
Mercy University
Dobbs Ferry, New York
Touro University
New York City, New York
Clinical Supervisor
Cerebral Palsy of Westchester
White Plains, New York

FOREWORD

I strongly believe that the use of theory as a tool for practice differentiates professionals from nonprofessionals. Although common sense has a place in decision making, professionals understand that many times our senses cannot be trusted. For example, if you are seated in a train car, your senses may give you the illusion that the trees and buildings outside the train are moving. However, you very well know that it is the train that is actually moving because you understand how the train is pulled by an engine so that it moves on wheels. You have a theoretical understanding of the mechanics of movement for a train. Therefore, you can disregard the illusion of your sense perception that the world around you is moving while you are stationary in a train. Put another way, as Drs. Laverdure and Seruya aptly state in this book, theory helps us explain the phenomena of interest in our experiences and make predictions based on that explanation.

Professions have theories that constitute bodies of knowledge that guide practitioners in decision making regarding matters of professional practice. Psychologists and psychotherapists have a variety of psychological theories (behaviorism, psychoanalysis, cognitive-behavioral theories, and so on) that guide how they work with their service users. The same thing is true for social workers, engineers, and so on. Occupational therapy practitioners should similarly be guided by theories that provide explanatory propositions about the definition of service users, issues in their domain of concern, and predictions of the effect of therapeutic interventions. Occupational therapy is grounded on the idea that human beings are occupational by nature and that occupational participation is necessary for health and well-being across the life span.

Occupational therapy practice is complex because many factors affect practitioners' attempts to provide high-quality services to facilitate meaningful occupational participation. In recent times, there has been an appropriate focus on evidence-based practice. This means that occupational therapy practitioners are called on to use interventions that are proven through research to be effective in creating change that enables service users to participate effectively in their meaningful daily occupations. However, evidence-based practice that is devoid of a clear application of the profession's theory can be problematic. It can lead to the use of presumably evidence-based interventions that lack fidelity to the profession's identity. Loss of identity could be a threat to the profession's existence in the long term.

Irrespective of where they practice, occupational therapy practitioners have to evaluate their service users (collect data) using well-validated assessments, use the evaluation information (data) to plan interventions that are supported by research evidence, and track the effectiveness of their treatment through a regular reassessment of outcomes. In this process, they have to take into account contextual factors that impact occupational performance. For example, in the school system, which is the focus of this book, some of the contextual factors include the Individuals with Disabilities Education Act and the related legal mandate to provide every student with a free appropriate public education in the least restrictive environment irrespective of disability. These contextual factors require that occupational therapy practitioners work effectively in teams with other professionals while ensuring their services are unique and valuable. Without using occupational therapy theory to guide decision making, it may be difficult to demonstrate the uniqueness and value of the services they provide. Drs. Laverdure and Seruya eloquently argue in this book that theoretical foundations help practitioners keep contextual factors in perspective so that they are appropriately oriented to practice that gives them their unique identity.

Drs. Laverdure and Seruya identify a problem: occupational therapy practitioners often do not value theory highly. Some of the reasons for this neglect of theory include its perceived irrelevance to issues of practice; lack of a good understanding of theory by the practitioners; and lack of structure for its application, especially given that no single theoretical framework on its own can adequately address all issues that come up in practice. Drs. Laverdure and Seruya contribute to the amelioration of this problem for occupational therapy practice in the school system by outlining guidelines for integrating theories in practice using frameworks such as Leclair's Theory Advancement Process and Ikiugu's eclectic method. These guidelines should be effective in promoting the uptake of theory by occupational therapy practitioners in the school system. Their effort in this endeavor is laudable, and similar guidelines should be developed for practitioners in all occupational therapy specialties. I hope readers find this work informative and practical as a guide to the use of theory as a tool for high-quality practice.

—Moses N. Ikiugu, PhD, OTR/L, FAOTA

FOREWORD

Theory is at the heart of what we do. When you watch an occupational therapist in practice, it looks like what we do is simple, but it is not. Evaluation and intervention are complex processes that are based in theory, the theories that we believe will successfully work and will bring about change in our students and clients. The strong basis of theory is what separates us from many other professions. It is not just something we teach students, but something we use every day in effective practice. I was first introduced to theory as a critical foundation of our profession during my graduate work at New York University, under Dr. Anne Cronin Mosey. Later, in the early 1990s, I began writing about the importance of theory to practice, particularly in pediatrics.

While theory has been around in the profession of occupational therapy for many years, Drs. Laverdure and Seruya and their contributors have explicitly brought it into the educational system and school-based practice with this book. As someone who started out as a novice working in the school system, I know this would have been an invaluable tool for me as a new therapist. This book ties together many critical areas of school-based practice: occupation, function, participation, health management, the importance of sleep, and how practice in the educational environment relates to our professional values. Even more important, it concentrates on the key areas that support sound theory-based practice: gathering data, evaluation, collaboration, and intervention. They raise the importance of mentoring, professional reasoning, and theory-based decision making. All are key to successful school-based practice.

School-based practice has been a growing area of employment for occupational therapy practitioners since the Education for All Handicapped Children Act in 1975 and has continued to grow with the Individuals with Disabilities Education Act (2004). I applaud the work that the authors have done here as I believe this book will be a major contribution for practitioners in the educational environment and a must have resource for those who teach this area of practice.

References

Education for All Handicapped Children Act, Pub. L. 94-142, 1975.
Individuals with Disabilities Education Act of 2004, Pub. L. 108-446, 20 U.S.C. §1400 et seq.

—Paula Kramer, PhD, OTR, FAOTA

INTRODUCTION

Occupational therapy practice that is guided by conceptual ideas of the meaning and value of occupation provides a systematic way to consider participation challenges, enables the identification of priorities for intervention to support successful participation, and helps us identify and articulate what we do and why we do it (Dunn, 2011; Kielhofner, 2009). The use of theoretical foundations in educational practice provides an essential scaffold to understand one's client within their occupational context. Additionally, the use of theory provides legitimacy to our professional concepts, especially the preeminence of occupation and of individuals as occupational beings. The use of conceptual constructs found within our theories allows us to define who we are as a profession as well as the ability to articulate our distinct value to the array of stakeholders who we interact with on our school teams and within our local, state, and federal educational agencies. The importance of theory has been echoed by many within the field (Ikiugu, 2007; Wong & Fischer, 2015), and theory plays a vital role in the education of practitioners. Theory-guided practice provides a scientifically based explanation developed to understand a specific phenomenon.

In this book, we consider theoretical foundations to be integrated collections of ideas and concepts that describe the relationships among them in a way that enables us to understand how things work and explain them to others; to test them both empirically and clinically; and, perhaps most relevant for practice, to be able to make predictions about what will happen and why. The profession has had a long history of changing theoretical orientations and paradigm shifts in response to contextual conditions such as our expanding knowledge, sociopolitical influences, and regulatory and economic requirements. In the profession's formative years, there was a focus on humanism and holistic engagement, but following the World Wars and in response to the alignment with the medical community, occupational therapy practitioners adopted medical and reductionist theoretical foundations that shifted focus to biomechanical, neuromuscular, and sensorimotor approaches that aligned with these societal needs to elevate and legitimize the profession. Today we see a return to occupation as the core construct of our profession, and our theoretical foundations have followed.

Occupational therapy practice in educational settings has likewise been influenced by sociopolitical, regulatory, professional, and scientific changes. Occupational therapy practitioners entered school practice in large numbers following the legislative changes that enabled public school access for students, even those with handicapping conditions. At that time, the profession was codifying and adopting frames of reference that guided restorative intervention, and our work in schools centered on addressing the needs of the most severely impaired students. Over the years, legislation and theoretical changes occurred in tandem, influencing where and how students with disabilities were educated, and occupational therapy service delivery gradually became increasingly client centered, occupation and participation focused, and evidence based.

Effective use of theoretical foundations in occupational therapy practice enables practitioners to align and synthesize observation, organize and unify data collection, frame and guide professional reasoning, scaffold the development of interventions and outcome measures, and guide analysis of intervention outcomes (Krefting, 1985; Steward, 1996; Wimpenny et al., 2010). Theory-based practice promotes the establishment of clear professional identity and a sense of evidence-based contribution; yet, research indicates that less than one quarter of occupational therapy practitioners regard theory to be of high value in their daily practice and the longer they work in a specific area of practice the less likely they are to rely on theory to guide practice (Bowen et al., 2005; Forsyth & Hamilton, 2005; Green, 2000; Ikiugu, 2010; O'Neal et al., 2007). The literature continues to suggest that practitioners do not thoroughly value, understand, or feel comfortable implementing theory-based interventions (Ikiugu, 2012; Lee et al., 2008; Nelson, 1996). Occupational therapy practitioners report a lack of understanding, tools, and resources for effective theory application; find theory too abstract and restrictive for use in practice; and indicate that no single approach is adequate in addressing occupational performance and participation. Although occupational therapy practitioners report these concerns regarding the application of theory to their practice, without theory guiding practice, we are often deprofessionalized and experience role identity confusion.

To fill the conceptual void and ground practice in a meaningful way, occupational therapy practitioners in school settings have long described their practice as conceptually grounded in an educational vs. medical model (Laverdure & Rose, 2012). We have "modelized" our thinking into a dichotomous medical vs. educational framework, valuing our contribution in addressing functional, developmental, and academic needs; determining educational disability; identifying adverse educational impact; and evaluating performance and progress in educational curriculum over knowledge of health, wellness, and participation. When we base our practice on our theoretical foundations, we more effectively balance our knowledge contributions and bring valuable scientific, pragmatic, interactive, narrative, and conditional reasoning skills and knowledge of child growth, developmental trajectories, and prognostication and become the team's central translators of knowledge of complex health, educational, and functional issues. In the absence of theoretical foundations in school practice, our professional reasoning may not be well formulated, evaluation may not be well aligned, intervention outcomes may not be adequately measured, and effective and efficacious service delivery may suffer (Laverdure & Rose, 2012). The educational vs. medical model dichotomy simply does not provide sufficient guidance to support effective professional reasoning and decision making. We need clear and intentional use of theory to support task performance, functional skill, and educational participation.

In this book, we address a critical need in the school-based occupational therapy practice community for a conceptual and pragmatic model of integrating theoretical foundations in practice. We aim to fill a critical gap in the translation and application of theory in occupational therapy practice in school-based settings, a gap that influences occupational therapy practitioner job satisfaction and effectiveness as well as system, family, and student outcomes. We propose a model derived from occupation-based conceptual models, the use of an organizing and complementary model framework (Ikiugu, 2012), and decision-making structures that aligns with educational requirements and supports collaborative and contextually designed evaluation and intervention. We examine the unique practice context of occupational therapy in educational settings and the requirements for collaborative decision making. We integrate the major evidence-based occupational therapy theoretical models and frames of reference that can be used effectively with children and youth to support the occupational therapy process and outcomes in educational settings. We provide explicit case examples of the implementation of these theoretical foundations and provide clear practice guidance on the implementation of a theory-guided occupational therapy process across school settings.

Throughout the book, we aim to cite primary sources of information addressing occupational therapy theory but apply it in contemporary ways that align with the American Occupational Therapy Association's *Occupational Therapy Framework: Domain and Process, Fourth Edition* (2020) and occupational therapy's ever-evolving evidentiary base. We additionally acknowledge that when current literature is available, we cite it; however, there remains scant research on the application of occupational therapy's body of theoretical knowledge in school-based practice. Therefore, this book also serves as a call for action for the examination, development, and implementation of theory and theory-based practice in school-based occupational therapy.

References

American Occupational Therapy Association. (2020). Occupational therapy practice framework: Domain and process (4th ed.). *American Journal of Occupational Therapy, 74*(Suppl. 2), 7412410010p1-741241001p87. https://doi.org/10.5014/ajot.2020.74S2001

Bowen, S., Martens, P., & Need to Know Team. (2005). Demystifying knowledge translation: Learning from the community. *Journal of Health Services Research and Policy, 10,* 203-211. https://doi.org/10.1258/135581905774414213

Dunn, W. (2011). *Best practice: Occupational therapy for children and families in community settings* (2nd ed.). SLACK Incorporated.

Forsyth, K., & Hamilton, E. (2005). Social service occupational therapists' view of practice and integration with health: A survey. *British Journal of Occupational Therapy, 71*(2), 64-71.

Green, J. (2000). The role of theory in evidence-based health promotion practice. *Health Education Research, 15*(2), 125-129.

Ikiugu, M. (2007). *Psychosocial conceptual practice models in occupational therapy: Building adaptive capability.* Elsevier.

Ikiugu, M. (2010). Analyzing and critiquing occupational therapy practice models using Mosey's extrapolation method. *Occupational Therapy in Health Care, 24*(3), 193-203. https://doi.org/10.3109/07380570903521641

Ikiugu, M. (2012). Use of theoretical conceptual practice models by occupational therapists in the US: A pilot study. *International Journal of Therapy and Rehabilitation, 19*(11), 629-637. https://doi.org/10.12968/ijtr.2012.19.11.629

Kielhofner, G. (2009). *Conceptual foundations of occupational therapy practice* (4th ed.). F. A. Davis.

Krefting, L. (1985). The use of conceptual models in clinical practice. *Canadian Journal of Occupational Therapy, 52*(4), 173-178. https://doi.org/10.1177/000841748505200402

Laverdure, P., & Rose, D. (2012). Educational relevance in school-based occupational and physical therapy. *Physical & Occupational Therapy in Pediatrics, 32,* 347-354.

Lee, S. W., Taylor, R., Kielhofner, G., & Fisher, G. (2008) Theory use in practice: A national survey of therapists who use the Model of Human Occupation. *American Journal of Occupational Therapy, 62*(1), 106-117. https://doi.org/10.5014/ajot.62.1.106

Nelson, D. (1996). Therapeutic occupation: A definition. *American Journal of Occupational Therapy, 50,* 775-782. https://doi.org/10.5014/ajot.50.10.775

O'Neal, S., Dickerson, A. E., & Holbert, D. (2007). The use of theory by occupational therapists working with adults with developmental disabilities. *Occupational Therapy in Health Care, 21*(4), 71-85. https://doi.org/10.1080/J003v21n04_04

Steward, B. (1996). The theory/practice divide: Bridging the gap in occupational therapy. *British Journal of Occupational Therapy, 59,* 264-268.

Wimpenny, K., Forsyth, K., Jones, C., Matheson, L., & Colley, J. (2010). Implementing the Model of Human Occupation across a mental health occupational therapy service: Communities of practice and a participatory change process. *British Journal of Occupational Therapy, 73*(11), 507-516. https://doi.org/10.4276/030802210X12892992239152

Wong, S. R., & Fischer, A. (2015). Comparing and using occupation-focused models. *Occupational Therapy in Health Care, 29*(3), 297-315. https://doi.org/10.3109/07380577.2015.1010130

A Model of Theory-Based Decision Making in School Practice

Patricia Laverdure, OTD, OTR/L, BCP, FAOTA
and Francine M. Seruya, PhD, OTR/L, FAOTA

Chapter Objectives

1. Describe the relationship of occupational therapy theoretical foundations and occupational therapy practice.
2. Examine occupational therapy practice in educational settings and identify the array of service delivery options available to support educational outcomes.
3. Compare and contrast the influence of educational systems' requirements and occupational therapy theoretical foundations on the provision of occupational therapy service delivery in educational settings.

Occupational therapy evaluation and intervention are guided by conceptual ideas of the meaning and value of occupation and its impact on health and wellness. These conceptual ideas, known in the occupational therapy literature as *theories, conceptual and practice models*, and *frames of reference (FOR)*, provide a "systematic way to consider participation problems and identify the priorities for intervention to support successful participation" (Dunn, 2011, p. 39). In addition, they underscore what occupational therapy practitioners do in their practice and why they do it (Kielhofner, 2006). Theories, conceptual and practice models, and FORs are, in fact, the sinew that connects observation, data synthesis, and analysis and supports the development of plausible hypotheses and intervention to enhance client access, participation, and belonging. Parham (1987) argues that effective

Laverdure, P., & Seruya, F. M. *Theory in School-Based Occupational Therapy Practice: A Practical Application* (pp. 1-11).
DOI: 10.4324/9781003526773-1

decision making in occupational therapy practice requires an explicit understanding of the profession's theoretical foundations. Without a thorough understanding of the profession's theoretical foundations, practitioners often lose their bearings as occupational therapy professionals and have difficulty articulating the value of their service in the lives of their clients (Ikiugu, 2010; Ikiugu & Smallfield, 2011; Parham, 1987; Schon, 1983).

Conceptual ideas guide occupational therapy practice across populations and context, and educational practice is no different. In this chapter, we examine the unique occupational therapy practice context and how the context influences educational settings and defines the occupations that occur within it. We identify the way in which theoretical foundations are situated in educational practice and discuss the ways in which occupational therapy practitioners use the profession's theoretical foundations to support decision making within this specialized context.

EDUCATION SETTING: A UNIQUE PRACTICE CONTEXT

The Educational Context

Practicing in the educational setting requires an understanding of the local, state, and national regulations that guide it; professional standards that define and support it; and local requirements that influence and shape it. In 1975, the United States enacted Public Law 94-142, the Education for All Handicapped Children Act (the precursor to the Individuals with Disabilities Education Act of 2004 [IDEA]), granting free appropriate public education to all students, including students with disabling conditions. The law requires states and municipalities to (a) identify students with disabilities and improve how they are to be educated; (b) evaluate the educational outcomes of the identification and education efforts; and (c) provide due process protections for students and families. Without question, the passage of this landmark legislation and its subsequent revisions have had an indelible and lasting impact on students with disabilities across the nation.

Nearly one quarter of practicing occupational therapists and occupational therapy assistants (23.2% and 20%, respectively) work in educational settings in the United States according to a recent salary and workforce survey conducted by the American Occupational Therapy Association (AOTA, 2020). Practicing in educational settings is complex and requires the synthesis of requirements and guidance from our profession (e.g., state practice acts, professional practice guidance [the fourth edition of the *Occupational Therapy Practice Framework: Domain and Process* (AOTA, 2020) and *Guidelines for Occupational Therapy Services in Early Intervention and Schools* (AOTA, 2017)], and requirements from federal and state statute and policy [Americans with Disabilities Act Amendments Act of 2008, Assistive Technology Act of 2004, Elementary and Secondary Education Act of 1965, Every Student Succeeds Act of 2015 (ESSA), Family Educational Rights and Privacy Act of 1974, IDEA, Rehabilitation Act Amendments of 2004, and Social Security Act of 1965]) and local school system policy. The roles and responsibilities of occupational therapy practitioners in the educational environment vary considerably and generally fall within the following two broad focus areas:

1. Individualized mandated services: The requirement for individualized mandated services is articulated expressly in IDEA. IDEA suggests that "Disability is a natural part of the human experience and in no way diminishes the right of individuals to participate in or contribute to society. Improving educational results for students with disabilities is an essential element of our national policy of ensuring equality of opportunity, full participation, independent living, and economic self-sufficiency for individuals with disabilities" (IDEA, 2004). Accordingly, IDEA

outlines the way in which services provided across an array of disciplines must be provided to ensure a child's access to, participation in, and benefit from a publicly provided educational program. Occupational therapy practitioners provide individualized mandated services to students in educational settings. Occupational therapy practitioners work with students and their caregivers to remove barriers to contexts and environments that preclude participation in activities that are natural and intended and to support participation that improves independent living, postsecondary education, and vocational outcomes. Additionally, services provided under the Rehabilitation Act Amendments of 2004 (Section 504) eliminate barriers that impede access to the educational contexts and environments and ensure accommodations to support participation in activities that are typical and intended.

2. School system–wide services: School system–wide services are articulated expressly in ESSA, and this comprehensive legislation ensures equal opportunity for all students in grades kindergarten through 12th grade. Under the guidance of ESSA, occupational therapy practitioners collaborate with school system administrators, teachers, staff, and caregivers to remove barriers that limit access to educational opportunities and improve learning contexts and environments for all students. School system–wide supports are largely described as tiered supports and are characterized by a comprehensive framework of resources and instruction to meet the needs of all students. Within this Multitiered System of Supports (often referred to as *Response to Intervention*), occupational therapy practitioners support the implementation of research-based principles and practices at three levels called *tiers* depending on the policy and procedure of the state educational agencies (SEAs) and local educational agencies (LEAs).

a. Tier 1: Provide high-quality standards-based education to all students by supporting programs, schools, and LEAs. By identifying and mitigating barriers to effective instruction and curricular and environmental access, occupational therapy practitioners ensure access to high-quality instruction for all students. Educative interventions that build capacity in teachers and staff to design curriculum, instruction and interventions that support all students, and advocacy for services and resources at the administrative level are common Tier 1 supports. Occupational therapy practitioners support the implementation of high-leverage educational practices through collaborative problem solving, modeling, and instruction (McLeskey et al., 2017).

b. Tier 2: Occupational therapy practitioners provide support and resources to teachers and staff to effectively meet the needs of subgroups of students who are not making adequate progress in the general education curriculum. This small group of students (approximately 5% to 15% of the population) may require supplemental resources beyond those provided at Tier 1 to accelerate their performance, and occupational therapy practitioners can bring unique resources and training to educational staff to enhance teaching and learning in the classroom for these groups. Depending on the regulations and policies of the SEA and LEA, occupational therapy practitioners may be involved in coinstructing students receiving Tier 2 supports.

c. Tier 3: Tier 3 interventions are reserved for those students who require the most significant support to make progress in the general education program (1% to 5% of the population). Once again, occupational therapy practitioners provide teachers and staff ways to design and implement instruction or adjust the environment to promote learning in this small group whose learning pace falls behind their grade-level peers or their learning style does not conform to the instructional practices offered to the larger classroom population. As mentioned previously, depending on the regulations and policies of the SEA and LEA, occupational therapy practitioners may be involved in coinstructing students receiving Tier 3 supports.

Whether individualized or school system–wide services are offered, occupational therapy practitioners examine the individual, the environment, and the typical and intended activities that occur within it and consider the influence of these factors on access, participation, and occupational performance. They make decisions based on the collected data and plan, provide, and measure the outcomes of interventions, and they support the life of the school and the inclusion of students within it. As a result, the client of the occupational therapy practitioner can be the student, caregivers, teachers, staff, school team, administrators, or the system as a whole.

Contextual Influences

Understanding the school context and the environmental and personal factors that define it is essential for success in the practice setting (AOTA, 2020). Context influences the student's participation and performance, the scope of the occupational therapy practitioner's contributions to the student's or the system's program, and the ways in which occupational therapy services are delivered and used (Muhlenhaupt, 2010). State and local educational and school policy and curriculum, student roles, responsibilities, routine and behavioral expectations, and internal (e.g., classroom and school) and external (e.g., community) characteristics influence the context of educational systems and must be considered when providing services. Establishing common language with educational professionals is essential. Understanding and using the language of educators and translating the language of occupational therapy and its theories, conceptual and practice models, and FORs to educational systems and their faculty and staff can help strengthen collaborative relationships that improve service delivery and outcomes.

Providing services in the educational context requires careful attention to the shifting public consensus, educational legislation, and judicial review. For example, the current educational statute prohibits school systems from denying a student an education because of their disability and from discrimination in identification and evaluation. Federal education law requires that school systems provide all students a free and appropriate education in the least restrictive environment, and it ensures that caregivers have the opportunity to participate in decisions regarding their child's educational program. Recent educational reforms mandate that (a) students with disabilities are educated in their neighborhood schools in regular classrooms with their nondisabled peers to the greatest extent as possible; (b) teams of educational professionals, specialists, and caregivers work together to evaluate educational access and learning, plan intervention, and collaboratively implement instruction using best available evidence; (c) expectations for progress are robust and evidence-based instruction, and interventions are delivered with fidelity; (d) progress is monitored collaboratively, outcomes are measured, and data are used to drive educational decision making; and (e) educational achievement, high school graduation, and employment rates rise among individuals with disabilities.

School provides students a unique opportunity to develop an understanding of their capabilities; establish identity and character; and form the roles and routines that will lead to satisfying engagement in independent living, postsecondary education, and vocational pursuits in their adult roles (Holahan et al., 2013). Bendixen and Kreider (2011) suggested that participation in school occupations provides students the opportunity to not only develop the skills for learning but also is an essential context for the development of self-expression, friendships, and belonging. Although the student's occupational profile changes across the life span, it is influenced by the roles, routines, and rituals they experienced at school. Occupational therapy practitioners use participation in activities of daily living and instrumental activities of daily living, education, work, play, leisure, rest, and social participation occupations to facilitate engagement across educational and extracurricular contexts

(Swinth, 2009). Occupational therapy practitioners are uniquely poised with understanding of the educational and extracurricular environment; the occupations, roles, and routines that occur within them; and how occupational performance is impacted by engagement in this dynamic context.

THEORIES, MODELS, AND FRAMES OF REFERENCE

A clear understanding of occupational therapy's theoretical foundations assists practitioners in identifying its domain within the practice environment and articulating its focus and distinct value within the practice context (Steward, 1996; Wimpenny et al., 2010). Theory provides recognition of the profession's value to populations and society, highlights its unique contributions, and provides identity and a sense of meaningful contribution for its members (Krefting, 1985). The use of theory in practice organizes and unifies data collection, aligns and synthesizes observation, frames and defines hypotheses, and scaffolds the development of interventions and outcome measures.

Although the field is widening, many of the theoretical foundations used by occupational therapy practitioners are undergirded by work done by other disciplines. The Accreditation Council for Occupational Therapy Education defines a theory as a "set of interrelated concepts used to describe, explain, or predict phenomena" (2018, p. 54). The phenomena described in theoretical foundations used in occupational therapy practice include (a) what effective engagement in occupation and occupational performance looks like, (b) the impact of dysfunction on occupational performance and participation, and (c) how to create change in occupational performance and enhance occupational participation. Some, although not all, occupational therapy applications of these theoretical foundations provide assessment tools, intervention resources and recommendations, and outcome measures.

In educational settings, theory guides the occupational therapy practitioner in answering two fundamental questions about the students they serve (Child Inclusion Research into Curriculum Learning Education Collaboration [CIRCLE], 2009): Who am I as a student? (What is the student's occupational identity?) and What can I do? (What is the student's occupational competence?).

The ways in which a student participates in school informs who they are and who they want to become. What the student finds interesting and important, who they interact with, and what they engage and feel effective engaging in defines their identity as an occupational being (CIRCLE, 2009). On the other hand, their occupational competence is defined by the ways in which the student "sustains a pattern of occupational participation that reflects identity" (CIRCLE, 2009, p. 10). Competence is observed in the way the student engages in and maintains engagement in occupations and routines that enable them to meet the expectations of their roles and their successful participation in occupations that enable satisfaction and fulfillment. Theoretical foundations in occupational therapy practice allow us to analyze the complexity of student occupational engagement.

Understanding Theories, Conceptual and Practice Models, and Frames of Reference

The fourth edition of the *Occupational Therapy Practice Framework: Domain and Process* (AOTA, 2020), an AOTA official document intended to summarize "interrelated constructs that describe occupational therapy practice" (p. 1), suggests that "Occupational therapy practitioners use theoretical principles and models, knowledge about the effects of conditions on participation, and available evidence on the effectiveness of interventions to guide their reasoning" (p. 1). Yet, distinction in the terms *theory, practice framework,* and *FOR* is often cloudy, and these terms may be used interchangeably in the occupational therapy literature. The inconsistent use of terms can cause considerable confusion when designing effective evaluation and intervention plans and articulating the value of occupational therapy services to stakeholders (Braveman & Kielhofner, 2006). Understanding the distinctions between them offers the occupational therapy practitioner a more effective way to access them and use them in practice.

A theory is, quite simply, a scientifically based explanation developed to understand a specific phenomenon. For example, we are driving along and a ball rolls into the road. Our knowledge and experience around balls rolling into the road informs an assumption that there is likely a child running behind the ball. In response to the pattern of understanding we have developed about balls rolling into the road, we apply the brakes, we look at the direction from which the ball came, and we scan the environment for confirmation of our prediction. Theory is the collection and analysis of a series of observations that are made and the formulation of a prediction or a hypothesis of what will happen given a particular action or circumstances. Hinojosa and colleagues (2010) suggested that when developing theories, we first observe an event or series of events (e.g., a ball rolling into the road). We describe the key phenomena, or the people, environment, and the events that take place within it, as concepts (e.g., the ball, road, car, driver, child). As patterns emerge, we begin to form causal relationships, called *postulates,* that help us conceptualize and categorize the concepts. A theory is formed from the relationship between the concepts and postulates (e.g., a ball rolling into the street is often followed by a running child). Conceptual models that guide our understanding of the student and their needs and address occupations, performance patterns, and contexts include occupation-based models such as the Person-Environment-Occupation-Performance model; the Model of Human Occupation; Synthesis of Child, Occupational, Performance, and Environment In Time; and activity engagement models.

As noted, occupational therapy draws its theory from a variety of disciplines, including its own, to define assumptions, concepts, and postulates in practice. Occupational therapy scholars and practitioners have used these broad conceptual ideas to form practice models and FORs. These practice models and FORs anchor specific concepts and postulates within a specific area of practice that enable occupational therapy practitioners to use theory predictably to define function, dysfunction, and mechanisms of change to gather relevant client data, design evaluation and intervention plans, and implement and evaluate intervention to effect change. In effect, given the characteristics of the client and their occupational performance challenges, when using a relevant theoretical approach, the occupational therapy practitioner can design intervention that with reasonable assurance will produce the expected outcome.

Commonly used practice models and FORs in occupational therapy practice include the following, which will be discussed in greater length in the following chapters:

- Practice models that support the development of intervention approaches that specifically address client factors and performance skills to include the following:
  - Biomechanical, motor learning, and sensory-based models
  - Neuroplastic, developmental, and acquisitional skill models
  - Ecological, learning, and public health models
  - Social and cognitive models
- Decision-making frameworks that guide professional reasoning in evaluation and intervention planning such as the following:
  - Intervention planning and implementation models (Occupational Therapy Intervention Process Model, Student-Environments-Tasks-Tools Framework, and Human Activity Assistive Technology Model)
  - Decision-making models (data-driven decision making)

Practice models and FORs provide additional organizing structures to examine and guide practice. Mosey (1981) suggested that there are six key elements of a model or FOR:

1. An underlying theoretical foundation: Core concepts and postulates that describe the observed phenomena
2. Philosophical assumptions: Core beliefs about function and dysfunction and how it impacts access and participation
3. Ethics: Expectations for the role of the practitioner in the formative and healing process of the client
4. A domain of concern: Areas of relevance to address through the occupational therapy process
5. Nature/principles for sequencing aspects of practice: Ways in which to address dysfunction and the mechanisms of change
6. Legitimate tools: The structure and process of intervention

USE OF THEORY IN PRACTICE

Despite the value of theories to practice, less than one quarter of occupational therapy practitioners regard theory to be of high value in their daily practice (O'Neal et al., 2007). Additionally, the longer one works in a specific area of practice, the less likely they are to rely on theory to guide their practice. Although theoretical foundations are a principal component in occupational therapy education programs and are required content by the accrediting body of the profession, the Accreditation Council for Occupational Therapy Education (2018), there are a number of factors that impede their use in practice. Cole and Tufano (2020) suggested that theoretical foundations, conceptual models, and FORs are often generated by academic scholars with little input from practitioners, limiting their relevance and applicability to clinical practice. Many occupational therapy practitioners either lack understanding of the applications of the profession's theoretical foundations or find them too abstract and restrictive for use in practice (Ikiugu, 2010; O'Neal et al., 2007). Additionally, Green (2000) reported that occupational therapy providers find that no single approach is adequate in addressing a client's occupational performance and participation. Many occupational therapy practitioners instead consider their use of theoretical foundations as eclectic, and they often combine a number of models without a specific structure or clear understanding to do so (Ikiugu, 2012). There is a paucity of knowledge translation models that support the application of theory to practice and the integration and application of theoretical foundations and scientific evidence (Bowen et al., 2005). Forsyth and Hamilton (2005) reported that occupational therapy practitioners often find technical skills more valuable to support decision making than theoretical principles.

Because of the pressures of productivity and accountability, occupational therapy practitioners who do not see an immediate application or benefit of the use of theoretical foundations in daily practice may not be inclined to invest the time it takes to keep abreast of changes within them (Law & McColl, 1989; Lee et al., 2008; O'Neal et al., 2007). A lack of evaluation and outcome measurement tools, client education resources, and intervention space and resources may limit their use in practice as well. Finally, theoretical foundations used by occupational therapy practitioners must be consistent with their values and the values and interests of the practice context to be used effectively in practice (Wimpenny et al., 2010) and be accepted by one's colleagues in order to be adopted and used consistently in clinical practice (McColl, 2000; O'Neal et al., 2007).

In a study of occupational therapy practitioners working with adults with developmental disabilities, researchers found that although practitioners often articulate the use of remedial theoretical approaches to include in their work with this population (sensory integration and biomechanical were among the most commonly cited approaches), they most often use compensatory approaches in their interventions with clients (O'Neal et al., 2007). Occupational therapy practitioners in school practice commonly report using Ayres Sensory Integration in their practice with students as well (Brown et al., 2009; Rodger et al., 2006) but have difficulty explaining concepts and factors of function, dysfunction, and change that influence student engagement and participation. Rarely do occupational therapy practitioners in schools use assessment and interventions that align explicitly with Ayres Sensory Integration approaches.

The number of occupation-based theories, conceptual and practice models, and FORs has grown rapidly over the last 3 decades (Lee, 2010). Towns and Ashby (2014) reported that occupational therapy practitioners who explicitly use occupation-based theory in practice engage clients more readily in occupations of meaning and exhibit strong professional identity and resilience. Conversely, those who do not ground their practice in occupation-based theory tend to frame their practice around performance components, designing evaluation and intervention from a bottom-up perspective and framing collaborative partnerships from a technical skills–based knowledge perspective. Deprofessionalization is common and is often expressed by occupational therapy practitioners as a loss of the ability to use the unique domain of occupational therapy to benefit students and ability to identify as an occupational therapy professional. In school practice, occupational therapy practitioners struggle with role identity and with articulating the value of the contributions made to students, families, and school teams.

CONCLUSION

The use of theoretical foundations in occupational therapy practice is vital; yet, it remains challenging for many practitioners (Ikiugu & Smallfield, 2011). There are few examples of strategies and processes that have effectively strengthened the capacity of occupational therapy practitioners to use them to guide decision making in practice (Leclair et al., 2013). Among the studies that have been conducted, researchers have found that the uptake and use of theoretical foundations to guide decision making improves when (a) occupational therapy practitioners understand the value of theoretical foundations and believe in the importance of theory to their practice (Boniface et al., 2008); (b) the theoretical foundations are consistent with the occupational therapy practitioner values and area of practice (Wimpenny et al., 2010); (c) focus is placed on building occupational therapy practitioner's knowledge, skills, and comfort with the use of theory (Keponen & Launiainen, 2008; Melton et al., 2010); and (d) a collaborative approach that offers opportunity for reflection and discussion is used to build the capacity of theory use (Boniface et al., 2008; Kielhofner, 2005a, 2005b; Wimpenny et al., 2010).

In the following chapters, we examine occupational therapy foundations commonly used in occupational therapy practice in school settings. We discuss the translation and application of theory in occupational therapy practice in school-based settings and provide a conceptual and pragmatic model of integrating theory-based decision making in school practice, a gap we believe influences occupational therapy practitioner job satisfaction and effectiveness as well as system, family, and student outcomes. We believe that the information presented provides an important blueprint for the advancement of occupational therapy practice in the context of educational reform and accountability. Leclair and colleagues (2013) examined the uptake and use of theoretical foundations in occupational therapy practice and established a collaborative model of theory advancement that we draw from in this text. The Theory Advancement Process was established as a "process of reflection and action that can be used to engage stakeholders to improve the relevance, uptake, and use of theory in occupational therapy practice" (Leclair et al., 2013, p. 186). The Theory Advancement Process identifies the following:

- Primary contexts that consider the client, practitioner, institution, and practice. In this book, we carefully identify our clients and the roles, responsibilities, and contributions of the occupational therapy practitioner in educational practice.
- A climate of collaborative relationships in which trust, power sharing, sensitivity, and respect are explicitly and openly examined and facilitated. We examine the influence of occupational therapy foundations on the collaborative decision-making structures of educational teams and how occupational therapy practitioners use theory to guide their actions in the consensus-based decision-making environment of educational teams.
- Essential processes that include building capacity, engaging in discourse, collaborating, and using theory with intention. Finally, we share a conceptual and pragmatic model of integrating theory-based decision making in educational practice settings.

REFERENCES

Accreditation Council for Occupational Therapy Education. (2018). Standards and interpretive guide. https://acoteonline.org/accreditation-explained/standards/

American Occupational Therapy Association. (2017). Guidelines for occupational therapy services in early intervention and schools. *American Journal of Occupational Therapy, 71*(Suppl. 2), 7112410010. https://doi.org/10.5014/ajot.2017.716S01

American Occupational Therapy Association. (2020). Occupational therapy practice framework: Domain and process (4th ed.). *American Journal of Occupational Therapy, 74*(Suppl. 2), 7412410010p1-7412410010p87. https://doi.org/10.5014/ajot.2020.74S2001

Americans with Disabilities Act Amendments Act of 2008, Pub. L. 110-325, 122 Stat. 3553 (2008).

Assistive Technology Act of 2004, Pub. L. 108-364, 118 Stat. 1707 (2004).

Bendixen, R. M., & Kreider, C. M. (2011). Review of occupational therapy research in the practice area of children and youth. *The American Journal Occupational Therapy, 65*(3), 351-359. https://doi.org/10.5014/ajot.2011.000976

Boniface, G., Fedden, T., Hurst, H., Mason, M., Phelps, C., Reagon, C., & Waygood, S. (2008). Using theory to underpin an integrated occupational therapy service through the Canadian model of occupational performance. *British Journal of Occupational Therapy, 71*(12), 531-539.

Bowen, S., Martens, P., & Need to Know Team. (2005). Demystifying knowledge translation: Learning from the community. *Journal of Health Services Research and Policy, 10*(4), 203-211. https://doi.org/10.1258/135581905774414213

Braveman, B., & Kielhofner, G. (2006). Developing evidence based occupational therapy programming. In B. Braveman (Ed.). *Leading and managing occupational therapy services* (p. 217). AOTA Press.

Brown, T., Rodger, S., Brown, A., & Roever, C. (2009). A profile of Canadian pediatric occupational therapy practice. *Occupational Therapy in Health Care, 21*(4), 39-69. https://doi.org/10.1080/J003v21n04_03

Child Inclusion Research into Curriculum Learning Education Collaboration. (2009). https://www.thirdspace.scot/wp-content/uploads/2021/02/Overview-of-CIRCLE-Resources-2021.pdf

Cole, M., & Tufano, R. (2020). *Applied theories in occupational therapy* (2nd ed.). SLACK Incorporated.

Dunn, W. (2011). *Best practice occupational therapy for children and families in community settings* (2nd ed.). SLACK Incorporated.

Elementary and Secondary Education Act of 1965, Pub. L. 89-10, 20 U.S.C. § 6301 et seq (1965).

Every Student Succeeds Act of 2015, Pub. L. 114-195, 114 Stat. 1177 (2015).

Family Educational Rights and Privacy Act of 1974, 20 U.S.C. § 1232g, 34 CFR Part 99 (1974).

Forsyth, K., & Hamilton, E. (2005). Social service occupational therapists' view of practice and integration with health: A survey. *British Journal of Occupational Therapy, 71*(2), 64-71.

Green, J. (2000). The role of theory in evidence-based health promotion practice. *Health Education Research,* *15*(2), 125-129.

Hinojosa, J., Kramer, P., & Luebben, A. (2010). Structure of the frame of reference. In P. Kramer & J. Hinojosa (Eds.), *Frames of reference for pediatric occupational therapy* (pp. 67-95). Lippincott Williams & Wilkins.

Holahan, L., Burton, S., Laverdure, P., & Muhlenhaupt, M. (2013). *Guidance for performance evaluation of* *school occupational therapists.* American Occupational Therapy Association. http://www.aota.org/-/media/ Corporate/Files/Practice/Children/Performance-Evaluation-School-based-Therapists10-31-13.pdf

Ikiugu, M. (2010). Analyzing and critiquing occupational therapy practice models using Mosey's extrapolation method. *Occupational Therapy in Health Care, 24*(3), 193-203. https://doi.org/10.3109/07380570903521641

Ikiugu, M. (2012). Use of theoretical conceptual practice models by occupational therapists in the US: A pilot study. *International Journal of Therapy and Rehabilitation, 19*(11), 629-637. https://doi.org/10.12968/ ijtr.2012.19.11.629

Ikiugu, M., & Smallfield, S. (2011). Ikiugu's eclectic method of combining theoretical conceptual practice models in occupational therapy. *Australian Occupational Therapy Journal, 58*(6), 437-446. https://doi. org/10.1111/j.1440-1630.2011.00968.x

Individuals with Disabilities Education Act of 2004, Pub. L. 108-446, 20 U.S.C. § 1400 et seq (2004).

Keponen, R., & Launiainen, H. (2008). Using the Model of Human Occupation to nurture an occupational focus in the clinical reasoning of experienced therapists. *Occupational Therapy in Health Care, 22*(2-3), 95-104. https://doi.org/10.1080/07380570801989549

Kielhofner, G. (2005a). Scholarship and practice: Bridging the divide. *American Journal of Occupational Therapy,* *59,* 231-239.

Kielhofner, G. (2005b). A scholarship of practice: Creating discourse between theory, research, and practice. *Occupational Therapy in Health Care, 19,* 7-16. https://doi.org/10.1300/J003v19n01_02

Kielhofner, G. (2006). *Research in occupational therapy: Methods of inquiry for enhancing practice.* F. A. Davis.

Krefting, L. (1985). The use of conceptual models in clinical practice. *Canadian Journal of Occupational Therapy,* *52*(4), 173-178. https://doi.org/10.1177/000841748505200402

Law, M., & McColl, M. A. (1989). Knowledge and use of theory among occupational therapists: A Canadian survey. *Canadian Journal of Occupational Therapy, 56,* 198-204.

Leclair, L. L., Ripat, J. D., Wener, P. F., Cooper, J. E., Johnson, L. A., Davis, E. L., & Campbell-Rempel, M. A. (2013). Advancing the use of theory in occupational therapy: A collaborative process. *Canadian Journal of Occupational Therapy, 80*(3), 181-193. https://doi.org/10.1177/0008417413495182

Lee, J. (2010). Achieving best practice: A review of evidence linked to occupation-focused practice models. *Occupational Therapy in Health Care, 24*(3), 206-222. https://doi.org/10.3109/07380577.2010.483270

Lee, S. W., Taylor, R., Kielhofner, G., & Fisher, G. (2008). Theory in practice: A national survey of therapists who use the Model of Human Occupation. *American Journal of Occupational Therapy, 62*(1), 106-117. https://doi. org/10.5014/ajot.62.1.106

McColl, M. A. (2000). Muriel Driver Memorial Lecture. Spirit, occupation and disability. *Canadian Journal of Occupational Therapy, 67*(4), 217-229. https://doi.org/10.1177/000841740006700403

McLeskey, J., Barringer, M.-D., Billingsley, B., Brownell, M., Jackson, D., Kennedy, M., Lewis, T., Maheady, L., Rodriguez, J., Scheeler, M. C., Winn, J., & Ziegler, D. (2017, January). *High-leverage practices in special education.* Council for Exceptional Children & CEEDAR Center.

Melton, J., Forsyth, K., & Freeth, D. (2010). A practice development programme to promote the use of the Model of Human Occupation: Contexts, influential mechanisms and levels of engagement amongst occupational therapists. *British Journal of Occupational Therapy, 73,* 549-558. https://doi.org/10.4276/03080221 0X12892992239350

Mosey, A. (1981). *Occupational therapy: Configuration of a profession.* Raven Press.

Muhlenhaupt, M. (2010). The perspective of context as related to frame of reference. In P. Kramer & J. Hinojosa (Eds.), *Frames of reference for pediatric occupational therapy* (pp. 67-95). Lippincott Williams & Wilkins.

O'Neal, S., Dickerson, A. E., & Holbert, D. (2007). The use of theory by occupational therapists working with adults with developmental disabilities. *Occupational Therapy in Health Care, 21*(4), 71-85. https://doi. org/10.1080/J003v21n04_04

Parham, D. (1987). Toward professionalism: The reflective therapist. *American Journal of Occupational Therapy,* *41,* 555-561. https://doi.org/10.5014/ajot.41.9.555

Rehabilitation Act Amendments of 2004, 29 U.S.C. §794 (2004).

Rodger, S., Brown, G. T., Brown, A., & Roever, C. (2006). A comparison of pediatrics occupational therapy university program curricula in New Zealand, Australia, and Canada. *Physical and Occupational Therapy in Pediatrics, 26*(1-2), 153-180.

Schon, D. A. (1983). *The reflective practitioner: How professionals think in action.* Basic Books.

Social Security Act of 1965, Pub. L. 89-97, 79 Stat. 286, Title XIX (2004).

Steward, B. (1996). The theory/practice divide: Bridging the gap in occupational therapy. *British Journal of Occupational Therapy, 59*, 264-268.

Swinth, Y. L. (2009). Evaluation of areas of occupation: Educational activities. In E. B. Crepeau, E. S. Cohn, & B. A. B. Schell (Eds.), *Willard and Spackman's occupational therapy* (11th ed., pp. 347-354). Wolters Kluwer Health/Lippincott Williams & Wilkins.

Towns, E., & Ashby, S. (2014). The influence of practice educators on occupational therapy students' understanding of the practical applications of theoretical knowledge: A phenomenological study into student experiences of practice education. *Australian Occupational Therapy Journal, 61*, 344-352. https://doi.org/10.1111/1440-1630.12134

Wimpenny, K., Forsyth, K., Jones, C., Matheson, L., & Colley, J. (2010). Implementing the Model of Human Occupation across a mental health occupational therapy service: Communities of practice and a participatory change process. *British Journal of Occupational Therapy, 73*(11), 507-516. https://doi.org/10.4276/030802210X12892992239152

2

Professional Identity
Owning Our Distinct Value

Francine M. Seruya, PhD, OTR/L, FAOTA
and Patricia Laverdure, OTD, OTR/L, BCP, FAOTA

Chapter Objectives

1. Describe the progression of state and federal educational regulation and policy and occupational therapy theoretical foundations since the passage of the landmark Education for All Handicapped Children Act of 1975.
2. Examine the internal and external influences that shape occupational therapy practice in school settings today.
3. Discuss the attributes of integrating both an educational and medical focus into our practice in school settings.
4. Compare and contrast professional identity and its reliance on theory-based practice.

The practice settings within which occupational therapy practitioners work are characterized by an array of specific regulatory, policy, and procedural considerations around which the scope of occupational therapy practice, clinical reasoning, and decision making must be integrated. Educational settings, as discussed in Chapter 1, are no different, and negotiating this practice setting requires that practitioners be aware of not only federal, state, and local regulatory statutes governing service provision and the policies and procedures that ensure compliance, but they must also develop a keen understanding of the social and political culture of the school and its system in which the policy is carried out. This chapter intends to briefly outline current practice patterns and trends within

Laverdure, P., & Seruya, F. M. *Theory in School-Based Occupational Therapy Practice: A Practical Application* (pp. 13-26). DOI: 10.4324/9781003526773-2

school-based practice, define and describe professional identity from a school-based perspective, and discuss how professional identity affects a practitioner's ability to apply their skills and knowledge in a manner that reflects current tenets of effective practice within schools.

PRACTICE PATTERNS AND TRENDS WITHIN SCHOOL-BASED PRACTICE

The Practice Context

The provision of services to children and youth in educational settings has changed considerably since the enactment of Public Law 94-142, the Education for All Handicapped Children Act (the precursor to the Individuals with Disabilities Education Act of 2004 [IDEA]) in 1975. Before its passage, children and youth lacked opportunities for education, and by 1969 it was estimated that more than 1 million children were excluded from educational opportunities (U.S. Department of Education [DOE], 2007). Children and youth who did receive services did so in state institutions for individuals with developmental disabilities or mental disorders, in hospitals or specialized clinics for children and youth with medical complexity (Muhlenhaupt, 2010), or supported through community-based programs such as the Association for Retarded Citizens and foundations such as Easterseals. Educational approaches used in these settings paid little heed to the students' chronological age, often used adapted curricular materials based on the students' mental age if any at all, and provided few developmental opportunities to fill the curriculum void. During the 1950s, occupational therapy practitioners slowly made their way into these settings, providing services along a medical continuum of care using biomechanical and recovery models that were the prevailing theoretical foundations of the time.

The 1960s and 1970s saw an expansion of social consciousness regarding civil rights across the country. Post–World War II breakthroughs in physical rehabilitation, neurology, and immunology brought about greater health care opportunities for individuals with long-term health issues and disabilities. At the same time, widespread efforts to recognize the civil rights of all, including those with disabilities, and deinstitutionalization of individuals with physical, developmental, and mental disabilities were underway, and community programs were overwhelmed with referrals for services. Armed with knowledge of valid approaches that improve the outcomes of children and youth with disabilities and fueled by the 1954 U.S. Supreme Court *Brown v. Board of Education of Topeka* case making segregation based on race unconstitutional, advocacy groups, including parents, occupational therapy practitioners, and the American Occupational Therapy Association (AOTA), endeavored to advance the rights of children and youth with disabilities to an appropriate education and establish educational and training opportunities at the local, state, and federal level. The following key provisions were enacted during that period (U.S. DOE, 2007):

- The Captioned Films Acts of 1958 (Public Law 85-905 and 85-926) and 1961 (Public Law 87-715) provided training materials for teachers of students with developmental disabilities.
- The Training of Professional Personnel Act of 1959 (Public Law 86-158) provided training to individuals to educate children and youth with developmental disabilities.
- The Teachers of the Deaf Act of 1961 (Public Law 87-276) provided training for instructional personnel for children and youth who were deaf or hard of hearing. It was later expanded to provide training across all disability categories (Public Law 88-164).
- The Higher Education Act (Public Law 88-204) and Maternal and Child Health and Mental Retardation and Facility Amendments (Public Law 88-156), both of 1963, supported the

advancement of curricular development, technical instruction, and community services for all students including children and youth with disabilities.

- The Elementary and Secondary Education Act (Public Law 89-10), now called the Every Student Succeeds Act (ESSA), and the State Schools Act (Public Law 89-313), both enacted in 1965, provided states with funding to support education for children and youth with disabilities. These critical provisions were among the first appropriated pieces of legislation designed to address the needs of students with disabilities and demonstrated federal commitment to provide educational improvements for educationally disadvantaged children.
- The Handicapped Children's Early Education Assistance Act of 1968 (Public Law 90-538) supported early childhood programs that provided needed resources for prevention and enrichment for children in need.

At the same time, advocacy groups continued to challenge the status quo in the courts in litigious efforts to expand equal access to educational opportunities for all students, including those with disabilities. Two of those cases used the Brown decision to specifically extend the right to educational opportunities to students with disabilities. In the first case, *Pennsylvania Association for Retarded Children (PARC) v. Commonwealth of Pennsylvania*, the Pennsylvania State Board of Education argued that it is relieved from providing educational services to students it deemed uneducable and untrainable and to those who had not achieved a mental age of 5 years (Forte, 2017). In their 1971 decision in favor of PARC, the District Court for the Eastern District of Pennsylvania laid the foundation for important provision in subsequent special education law to include the following:

- All students are capable of benefiting from an educational program.
- A free, public program of education and training appropriate to the child's capacity must be provided.
- Placement in a regular school is preferable to placement in a special school class or program.
- No change in a student's educational program can be made without notification and opportunity for due process.

The following year, in *Mills v. Board of Education of District of Columbia*, the school board argued that although it recognized the obligation to educate students capable of benefiting from instruction, it was incapable of doing so because it lacked sufficient funding (Forte, 2017). The court in this case decided again in favor of the plaintiff, indicating that a state educational agency (SEA) or local educational agency (LEA) could not deny a student an education based on insufficient funds. Twenty-seven additional federal court cases followed the PARC and Mills decisions leading to the landmark 1975 Education for All Handicapped Children Act (now called IDEA), which codifies the right to a free appropriate public education (FAPE) for all, including those with disabilities according to the following provisions:

- Schools receiving federal funds must provide access to educational opportunities to all students (FAPE).
- SEAs and LEAs must identify students with special needs (Child Find).
- Students must be provided an individualized program of education (Individualized Education Program) within the least restrictive environment.
- Students and their caregivers must be provided an opportunity to participate in education planning and decision making, and safeguards must be in place to ensure their rights (due process).
- Procedures, processes, and materials used to evaluate students must not discriminate based on student diversity factors (i.e., race, ethnicity, language, or sex).

Service Expansion

As services expanded for children and youth with disabilities, occupational therapy practitioners gradually gained a foothold across the range of service delivery systems that were supporting them and their needs, including public school settings. Students with severe physical disabilities were considered eligible and referred for occupational therapy services (Muhlenhaupt, 2010), and occupational therapy practitioners began to shift their knowledge and expertise developed in medical settings, such as hospital and specialty treatment centers, and apply it to service delivery in schools. These practice patterns prevailed until the range of students and their needs began to expand in the late 1980s and early 1990s. With our profession's expanding knowledge of neuroscience, occupational therapy practitioners began to recognize the value that occupational therapy services could add to the educational programs of students with intellectual disabilities and cognitive and perceptual social needs. In addition, the prevalence of students with autism spectrum disorders was increasing, and referrals for occupational therapy services multiplied. Occupational therapy practitioners gradually expanded their theoretical lens but continued to situate it largely within a focus on remediating disability, relying heavily on knowledge of biomechanics and neurology and aligning treatment on skills such as handwriting and sensory processing and modulation.

In addition to focusing on the remediation of performance skills, occupational therapy practitioners also used service delivery models that were similar to those used in hospital or outpatient settings. Typical practice included retrieving a student from their classroom, bringing them to a separate area, performing therapy services, and returning the child to the classroom. This professional reasoning and service delivery mirrored professional education and identity at that time (Cole & Tufano, 2019). Bringing students for individual or group therapy sessions in the therapy room to address underlying skill development such as intrinsic hand strength, scanning, and sensory processing became the typical model of occupational therapy in school-based settings (Spencer et al., 2006).

Although the overarching theoretical foundation continued to be medically based and reductionistic (Cole & Tufano, 2019) for some time, theoretical approaches were expanding across the health care, social and psychological, and educational spectrum, and occupational therapy conceptual models and frames of reference began to diversify. Although these models continued to situate heavily on biomechanical foundations, they included approaches such as neurodevelopmental, reflex, and voluntary movement and motor control approaches. Occupational therapy theory development was slowly being influenced by advancements in the fields of social psychology, cognitive, and learning, and by the early 1990s, occupational therapy practitioners slowly began introducing developmental, acquisitional, and task-oriented approaches to their work with children and youth; yet, handwriting and sensory processing and modulation remained its niche practice domains in school practice.

The Internal and External Influences on School Practice

Like the 1960s and 1970s, the 1990s and 2000s brought significant advancements in the provision of occupational therapy services for students in public school settings. School occupational therapy practice during that time was influenced by numerous social, political, and professional factors. First, during that period of time, the social view of disability began to shift. With the development and dissemination of the *International Classification of Functioning, Disability and Health (ICF)*, in 2000 the World Health Organization (2002) outlined a standard language and framework to describe health and health-related states. In a dramatic shift from previously articulated models of health and disability that largely shaped our understanding of disability as anatomic, physiologic, or mental abnormalities of organs or body systems and focused our attention on function of tissues, organs, and body systems, the *ICF* enabled us to view function as the result of a student's characteristics and attributes and the occupations, roles, routines, and environments in which they engage. The *ICF* shifts our focus from the things the student can and cannot do and places it on the ways in which the student participates in the occupations and activities that are typical given the student's age and grade level. Occupational therapy practitioners began to focus not only on the factors within the individual but also the occupations they pursue and the environments they pursue them in as influencing factors to effective function. In school settings, occupational therapy practitioners began to think about intervention not only from the perspective of remediation but also of how remediation in combination with education, accommodation, and modification could improve the student's participation in their educational program. An idea that there was a distinction between the way services were being delivered in schools vs. traditional medical settings began to take hold.

A second influencing factor was the continued call for the inclusion of all students, including those with disabilities, in educational opportunities provided in public schools (Lipsky & Gartner, 2012). Hansen and Hinojosa (1999) asserted that "Inclusion requires that we ensure not only that everyone is treated fairly and equitably, but also that all individuals have the same opportunities to participate in the naturally occurring activities of society, such as attending social events, access to public transportation, and participating in professional organizations" (p. 598). Advocacy groups and practitioners alike collaborated to create inclusive social, cultural, and physical environments in which active participation and social interaction of all children were emphasized and differences acknowledged and celebrated in order to enable students the opportunity to build the necessary skills for community belonging and self-advocacy that generalize to other communities and last throughout the life span (Shogren et al., 2015). Occupational therapy practitioners "equipped to identify the social participation needs of students with disabilities, describe the influence of supports and barriers on participation in meaningful and valued occupation, and prioritize interaction based upon the student's, family's, and teacher's goals and desired outcomes" (Laverdure et al., 2019, p. CE5) began to frame school practice patterns around promoting school access to the environments and the occupations that occur within them and the facilitation of social participation.

All while still using theoretical models that focused on client factors and performance skills, occupational therapy practitioners began to assess the influence of supports for and barriers to participation in meaningful and valued occupations and prioritize goals of the student, family, and teacher. With few theoretical tools to work with, school practitioners began designing student-centered interventions that consider personal and contextual factors that facilitate or interfere with participation in the educational experience (Başu et al., 2004). At the educational planning table, if not yet in service delivery, occupational therapy practitioners began to advocate for educational opportunities for peer-to-peer connection, choice making, and self-determination in the context of everyday activities across educational environments. As we grappled with the implementation of inclusive practices, we more fully embraced our unique role in an educational setting.

A third influencing factor aligned with the changes that were taking place in special education as a result of the serial reauthorizations and gradual alignment of key federal educational regulations, including IDEA and ESSA. As noted previously, IDEA ensures that all students with disabilities have access to a FAPE that emphasizes special education and related services designed to meet their unique needs and prepare them for further education, employment, and independent living (IDEA, 2004). ESSA requires that all students be taught to challenging academic content standards that prepare them to succeed in college and careers (English et al., 2017). The reauthorizations and alignment in these two bills emphasized the notion that the purpose of a student's educational experience in public school is to ensure their successful participation in the valuable adult occupations of independent living, education, and work.

Furthermore, in the early 2000s, the U.S. DOE introduced accountability measures to evaluate not only an SEA's and LEA's compliance with regulatory mandates but also their achievement of its purpose. In other words, are we not only effective at complying with procedures and procedural timelines, but are students making progress in their educational programs; graduating; transitioning to postschool living, educational, and vocational opportunities; and leading successful lives? Although many occupational therapy practitioners still primarily provide interventions in our niche practice domains of handwriting and sensory processing and modulation, many others have leveraged these changes to establish school-wide programs that support school climate and safety, student engagement, and postsecondary readiness; expand teacher capacity to meet the diverse instructional and social emotional needs of students; and participate in transition planning and development of postsecondary goals in the areas of training, education, employment, and independent living skills. Pressures to consider the long-term outcomes for students and prognosticate their educational trajectory solidified a conceptualization that there is a difference between the types of services one would provide in a medical setting (medical model) and those that would be provided in an educational one (educational model). However, the challenge for many of us is that there remains no theoretically distinguishable or assessed occupational therapy educational model around which to frame evaluation and intervention in the school setting.

Finally, a fourth factor to influence school occupational therapy practice in the 1990s and 2000s comes from the profession itself. In the early 1960s, Mary Reilly (1962) proposed that occupational therapy is one of the greatest ideas of the 20th century. It would take nearly 20 years of research on the nature of occupation, humans as occupational beings, and occupation's connection to health and well-being for the threshold concept of occupation to take root (Fortune & Kennedy-Jones, 2014; Sadlo, 2016). In 1998, 3 years before the word *occupation* was introduced once again in the official language of the profession, Nielson (1998) argued that occupational therapy programs must graduate students who deeply understand occupation and who can meaningfully translate it in practice. Later that year, Yerxa (1998) called for a professional renaissance of occupational therapy, identifying occupation as the central organizing idea. Yerxa suggested that individuals, in their "marvelous complexity and diversity" (p. 367), cannot be understood through a conceptual reduction below the level of the individual. The renaissance that Nielson and Yerxa speak of challenges occupational therapy practitioners, educators, and scholars to identify and examine approaches that not only enhance health and well-being but also distinguish the profession and effectively meet society's needs. The renaissance places occupation at the center of human experience in a global, technological postmodern world and situates individuals as occupational beings and occupational engagement as health promoting (Whiteford & Wilcock, 2001).

As the profession returned to an occupation-based philosophy (AOTA, 2017) and incorporated occupation as its core construct in documents such as the fourth edition of the *Occupational Therapy Practice Framework: Domain and Process* (AOTA, 2002, 2008, 2014b, 2020), there likewise was a shift in ideology within school-based practice. In 2017, the AOTA published "Guidelines for Occupational Therapy Services in Early Intervention and Schools" indicating that effective practice within schools should take place within natural settings to support the centralizing provisions of IDEA of FAPE, least restrictive environment, and students' participation and long-term outcomes. To achieve this end, the profession has advocated for contextually based, integrated service delivery models; yet, a nonintegrated, pullout model of service delivery continues to be a primary service delivery model used in current practice (Seruya & Garfinkel, 2020).

Because of the void of effective models to guide practice in educational settings, occupational therapy practitioners have begun to expand practice and use more contextually based service delivery structures. Instead of removing students from the classroom to provide services in a different location, the emphasis on classroom-based, contextually relevant service delivery is slowly taking hold. Occupational therapy practitioners are (a) exploring ways to embed services across settings to include the classroom, on the playground, and in the cafeteria to meet the needs of students (AOTA,

2014a; Frolek Clark & Chandler, 2013; Handley-More et al., 2013; Seruya & Garfinkel, 2018); (b) developing ways to collaborate with teachers that not only support the student but also build capacity in teachers to meet the instructional needs of students with disabilities (Laverdure, 2018; Laverdure et al., 2017); (c) providing whole-school and multitiered support services (Grajo et al., 2020; Handley-More et al., 2019); and (d) re-examining service delivery models from a caseload (the practitioner's day is determined by the number of students and associated treatment sessions mandated by Individualized Education Program minutes) to a workload model (the practitioner accounts for all of the workload responsibilities across everyday practice; Garfinkel & Seruya, 2018; Polichino & Jackson, 2014).

Once practitioners began providing services within classrooms, they more readily established collaborative relationships with teachers and classroom staff. However, providing contextually based services offers new challenges to the profession, and there remains confusion on how to implement skilled, professional services within classroom settings (Seruya & Garfinkel, 2018). It appears practitioners have difficulty explaining the rationale for their services within classroom settings and feel ill equipped to address skills from an occupation-based lens (Watt & Gage Richards, 2016). Practitioners began to reframe their services by reappropriating the rationale for their current goals rather than reframing the professional reasoning process (Kaplan & Seruya, 2019). For example, working on underlying skills for handwriting supported a child in their role of student and facilitated their ability to complete the occupation of completing written lessons. While embracing a model that favors the promotion of inclusive participation, once again occupational therapy practitioners in school practice rely on models that are antithetical to the influencing shifts in occupational therapy practice, leaving a foundational void in school practice.

EDUCATIONAL VERSUS MEDICAL MODEL

To fill the conceptual void and ground practice in a meaningful way, occupational therapy practitioners in school settings have long described their practice as conceptually grounded in an educational vs. medical model. The dichotomy may seem fitting because interdisciplinary educational teams are explicitly charged by IDEA to identify and address relevant functional, developmental, and academic needs that can support the determination of whether a student has an educational disability; whether that disability adversely affects the student's participation, performance, and progress in the general education curriculum; and whether the student requires specially designed instruction to access and make progress in their educational program (Jackson, 2007). Furthermore, as members of the team, occupational therapy practitioners collaboratively design and implement services and supports required for students to be successful in school (IDEA, 2004). Yet, occupational therapy practitioners are often central translators of knowledge of the complex medical, developmental, psychosocial, and emotional characteristics and provide valuable insights of the interactions of these characteristics on students' health, well-being, and participation in occupations and communities of meaning.

Team decisions regarding the provision of services in educational settings require the "synthesis of health-related parameters of the student (health conditions, body function and structures, and environmental context) and the educational trajectories and transitions that define the student's pathway through his or her educational process" (Laverdure & Rose, 2012, p. 348). In many cases, occupational therapy practitioners may be a student's and family's entry point to health care. Identifying health-related concerns often warrants referral to appropriate health care providers. Navigating care follow-up, integrating medical care plans, and translating the impact of medical conditions, precautions, and medications on learning and participation are critical roles of occupational therapy practitioners (Laverdure & Rose, 2012). Occupational therapy practitioners possess valuable scientific, pragmatic, interactive, and conditional reasoning skills that are, in fact, critical collaborative deci-sion-making assets that enable the team to effectively design evaluation and intervention plans in the educational setting (Schell & Schell, 2008).

Without a clear understanding and use of theoretical foundations in occupational therapy prac-tice, professional reasoning may not be well formulated, evaluation may not be well aligned, and interventions may not be adequately measured to ensure effective and efficacious service delivery (O'Neal et al., 2007). Occupational therapy practitioners build collaborative partnerships with fami-lies and school teams to strengthen capacity to support the education and engagement of students in meaningful occupation and communities; they empower students' increasingly independent de-cision-making capacity, efficacy, and responsibility to themselves and their communities; they look beyond disability and disease and consider the affordances and barriers that affect participation; and they facilitate active engagement in inclusive and collaborative communities.

IDEA, practice guidance, and the expanding body of research in occupational therapy interven-tion challenge practitioners to work toward the development of "a culture of universal accessibility and inclusivity in which active participation and social interaction of all children is emphasized and differences acknowledged and celebrated" (Laverdure & Rose, 2012, p. 353). The educational vs. medical model dichotomy no longer provides sufficient guidance to support effective professional reasoning and decision making in school practice. Instead, a theoretically grounded perspective is necessary as "a way of seeing clients, their impairments, their occupational circumstances, and their interpersonal characteristics" (Kielhofner, 2009, p. 281). This perspective, grounded in clear and intentional use of theories, conceptual and practice models, and frames of reference to support both student engagement in occupations and authentic belonging to communities of meaning and school cultures of universal accessibility and inclusivity, requires acknowledgment that there is more than one way to approach evaluation and intervention planning.

Using the occupation-based theories and models of practice provides guidance in the use of multiple and theoretically diverse approaches to address the needs of clients within unique and com-plex contexts (Hinojosa & Kramer, 2017). It underscores the need to continually evolve with the profession's expanding science; the context's shifting focus and priorities; the occupational therapy practitioner's knowledge and skill; and the client's evolving interests, values, and needs (Hinojosa & Kramer, 2017). This perspective does not eliminate or value one theoretical concept over another; instead, it enables occupational therapy practitioners the options to choose all available theoretical approaches that support student occupational engagement and community participation. We argue, in fact, that the contributions of occupational therapy practitioners in schools should be based on oc-cupational therapy theoretical foundations, however weakly they are articulated, vs. an educational or medical model that provides little meaning or context to the process or outcome of occupational therapy practice. The use of theoretical models is essential in that they provide the foundation for practitioners to understand their client within their occupational context. Additionally, the use of theory provides legitimacy to our core professional concepts, especially the preeminence of occupa-tion and people as occupational beings. The use of conceptual constructs found within our theory allows us to define who we are as a profession as well as the ability to articulate to consumers and stakeholders our distinct contribution to the educational team. The importance of theory has been echoed by many within the field (Ikiugu, 2007; Wong & Fischer, 2015) and plays a significant role in the education of practitioners. However, the literature continues to indicate practitioners do not thoroughly understand nor do they feel comfortable implementing theory-based practice in their day-to-day work (Ikiugu, 2012; Lee et al., 2008; Nelson, 1996).

PROFESSIONAL IDENTITY IN SCHOOL-BASED PRACTICE

Developing a professional identity begins within the academic setting. In their educational program, occupational therapy students learn the values and ethical principles of the profession and how these tenets fit in with their professional practice. Ikiugu and Rosso (2003) postulated that professional identity is strongly related to students' understanding of the theoretical underpinnings of the profession. Pierce (2001) and Wilcock and Townsend (2000) argued the necessity of establishing a strong philosophical base driven by theory to strengthen the identity of the profession. Students' enculturation into the profession continues with fieldwork placements. Each placement further facilitates a student's understanding of the norms and typical practice patterns as well as the professional reasoning processes used in practice settings. A new graduate from an entry-level academic program possesses the skills and knowledge of a generalist practitioner with a broad appreciation of the various settings within which occupational therapists practice. As an individual continues their practice, they continue to develop their personal and professional identity and become enculturated within their respective specialties and practice settings.

Occupation as a Core Construct

Studies indicate that individuals must possess a firm professional identity to successfully engage in interprofessional practice, and as practitioners move their practice to be more contextually relevant, interprofessional collaboration is an essential component of practice (Seruya & Garfinkel, 2018). The literature continues to indicate that occupational therapy practitioners and students often have difficulty articulating the meaning of occupation (Aiken et al., 2011; Seruya & Ellen, 2015; Smith & Mackenzie, 2011) and the need to strengthen entry-level therapists' professional identity (Howell, 2009). The literature is rife with varying definitions and examples of the meaning of occupation. A sampling of exemplars include the following:

- Occupation is the "essential current that propels each of us along on life's journey ... the occupations of our lives and the meanings of those occupations are essential contributors to the pace and direction of the life flow. Occupation is a powerful source of meaning in our lives; meaning arises from occupation and occupation arises from meaning" (Hasselkus, 2011, p. 21).
- "Occupation is everything people do to occupy themselves, including looking after themselves ... enjoying life ... and contributing to the social and economic fabric of their communities" (Law et al., 1998, p. 81).
- Occupations are "Daily activities that reflect cultural values, provide structure to living, and meaning to individuals; these activities meet human needs for self-care, enjoyment, and participation in society" (Crepeau, 2003, p. 190). They are "goal-directed pursuits that typically extend over time, have meaning to the performer, and involve multiple tasks" (Christiansen et al., 2005, p. 548). They involve "mental abilities and skills and may or may not have an observable physical dimension" (Hinojosa & Kramer, 1997, p. 865). They are the "chunks of daily activity that can be named in the lexicon of the culture" (Zemke & Clark, 1997, p. vii).
- "Occupation is used to mean all of the things people want, need, or have to do, whether of physical, mental, social, sexual, political, or spiritual nature and is inclusive of sleep and rest. It refers to all aspects of actual human doing, being, becoming, and belonging. The practical, everyday medium of self-expression or of making or experiencing meaning, occupation is the activist element of human existence whether occupations are contemplative, reflective, and meditative or action based" (Wilcock & Townsend, 2014, p. 542).

Although there is an appreciation for the diversity and varied perspectives the profession has embraced regarding the definition of our core construct of occupation, this same variability allows for ambiguity and makes it difficult for practitioners to articulate what it is we do as occupational therapists. We summarize these complex ideas, suggesting that occupations are the things that individuals, communities, and populations choose or need to participate in in order to engage fully and meaningfully in life roles and routines. It is important to note that, for the purposes of this text, we make a distinction between occupation and activity. In school practice, we share a common nomenclature with team members that we use to describe the activities that students are involved in (e.g., collecting food items on one's tray is an activity, an idea held in the minds of persons and in their shared cultural language; Pierce, 2001). An activity, although culturally defined and easily described and understood among team members, is not uniquely experienced by an individual and is not located in a fully existent temporal, spatial, and sociocultural context. Descriptions of activities enable us to communicate about occupational experiences in broad and accessible ways. On the other hand, occupations are a "specific individual's personally constructed, non-repeatable experience" (Pierce, 2001, p. 139). They are subjective, temporal, spatial, and sociocultural; have an infinite number of perceived contextual qualities; and have specific meaning that is fully known only to the individual engaged in the occupation (Dickie et al., 2006; Pierce, 2001). We are attentive then to the student's unique experience of gathering their food item on the tray in the context of personal factors and performance skills; the noisy and crowded cafeteria line; being surrounded by their classmates; and the sociocultural experience of eating lunch in that time, space, and setting.

Application of Identity in Practice

Possessing a strong professional identity allows individuals to be more effective, articulating not only what they do but why they do it. Therefore, practitioners who are able to articulate the core constructs of occupational therapy are better equipped to provide contextually based services because they are able to differentiate themselves from other professionals in the classroom and they are also able to offer professional reasoning and judgment aligned with theoretical concepts. Additionally, strong professional identity provides professionals with the ability to advocate for themselves (Ikiugu & Rosso, 2003).

Studies of practice patterns of school-based occupational therapy practitioners have indicated that practitioners continue to use individual services in a context other than the classroom such as a therapy room as their primary means of service provision in school settings (Spencer et al., 2006; Seruya & Garfinkel, 2020); yet, guidelines for effective practice in school settings state service delivery within contextually relevant settings lead to improved outcomes. Although there appears to be an incongruence, little attention has been relegated to how professional identity mediates a practitioner's ability to work collaboratively in contextually based settings such as the classroom.

The ability to reason and use theory as a means of professional identity and to substantiate the distinct value of who we are within the setting is a necessity. Practitioners cannot implement effective, contextually based models without the foundational theoretical constructs to support their clinical decision making and interventions. Likewise, the lack of theory base may facilitate the desire to continue implementing nonintegrated, pullout models of service delivery. Advocating and negotiating for increased presence in multitiered service models will require practitioners to be able to use foundational and theoretical constructs to support their distinct value within the school setting. Therefore, the need for a professional reasoning and decision-making framework appears to be warranted to facilitate the use of theoretical models and frameworks in school-based practice. Additionally, practitioners appear to need practical examples of how these models and frames would be appropriately implemented within a school setting to facilitate participation, inclusion, and occupational balance.

CONCLUSION

In this chapter, we examined the integrally connected links between sociopolitical policy, the progression of state and federal educational regulation, and occupational therapy theoretical foundations since the passage of the landmark 1975 Education for All Handicapped Children Act. Concepts of ability/disability and function shifted as the World Health Organization developed and updated the *ICF*. Likewise, occupational therapy's theoretical base shifted as a result of internal and external influences to form a holistic and participatory consensus of function as the result of a student's characteristics and attributes and the occupations, roles, routines, and environments in which they engage. We examined the shape of occupational therapy practice and the identity of occupational therapy practitioners in school settings today and considered the attributes of integrating both an educational and medical focus to our practice in school settings. Theoretical foundations and the use of them in practice, we argued, undergird our professional identity and guide how occupation, when framed as a central construct of the profession, promotes professional identity and supports the effective articulation of our distinct value to students, teams, schools, and school districts. In the coming chapters, we examine how theoretical foundations guide the domain and process of occupational therapy.

REFERENCES

Aiken, F. E., Fourt, A. M., Cheng, I. K. S., & Polatajko, H. J. (2011). The meaning gap in occupational therapy: Finding meaning in our own occupation. *Canadian Journal of Occupational Therapy, 78*, 294-302. https://doi.org/10.2182/cjot.2011.78.5.4

American Occupational Therapy Association. (2002). Occupational therapy practice framework: Domain and process. *American Journal of Occupational Therapy, 56*, 609-639. https://doi.org/10.5014/ajot.56.6.609

American Occupational Therapy Association. (2008). Occupational therapy practice framework: Domain and process (2nd ed.). *American Journal of Occupational Therapy, 62*, 625-683. https://doi.org/10.5014/ajot.62.6.625

American Occupational Therapy Association. (2014a). Occupational therapy's commitment to nondiscrimination and inclusion. *American Journal of Occupational Therapy, 68*, S23-S24. https://doi.org/10.5014/ajot.2014.686S05

American Occupational Therapy Association. (2014b). Occupational therapy practice framework: Domain and process (3rd ed.). *American Journal of Occupational Therapy, 68*(Suppl. 1), S1-S48. https://doi.org/10.5014/ajot.2014.682006

American Occupational Therapy Association. (2017). Philosophical base of occupational therapy. *American Journal of Occupational Therapy, 71*(Suppl. 2), 7112410045. https://doi.org/10.5014/ajot.716S06

American Occupational Therapy Association. (2020). Occupational therapy practice framework: Domain and process (4th ed.). *American Journal of Occupational Therapy, 74*(Suppl. 2), 7412410010p1-7412410010p87. https://doi.org/10.5014/ajot.2020.74S2001

Basu, S., Jacobson, L., & Keller, J. (2004). Child-centered tools: Using the Model of Human Occupation framework. *School System Special Interest Section Quarterly, 11*(2), 1-4.

Christiansen, C., Baum, M. C., & Bass-Haugen, J. (Eds.). (2005). *Occupational therapy: Performance, participation, and well-being.* SLACK Incorporated.

Cole, M., & Tufano, R. (2019). *Applied theories in occupational therapy* (2nd ed.). SLACK Incorporated.

Crepeau, E. (2003). Analyzing occupation and activity: A way of thinking about occupational performance. In E. Crepeau, E. Cohen, & B. Schell (Eds.), *Willard and Spackman's occupational therapy* (pp. 189-202). Lippincott.

Dickie, V., Cutchin, M., & Humphry, R. (2006). Occupation as transactional experience: A critique of individualism in occupational science. *Journal of Occupational Science, 13*(1), 83-93. https://doi.org/10.1080/14427591.2006.9686573

Elementary and Secondary Education Act of 1965, Pub. L. 89-10, 20 U.S.C. § 6301 et seq (1965).

English, D., Cushing, E., Therriault, S., & Rasmussen, J. (2017). *College and career readiness begins with a well-rounded education: Opportunities under the Every Student Succeeds Act.* American Institutes for Research, College and Career Readiness and Success Center.

Forte, J. (2017). *History of special education: Important landmark cases.* Forte Law Group, LLC. http://www.fortelawgroup.com/history-special-education-important-landmark-cases/

Fortune, T., & Kennedy-Jones, M. (2014). Occupation in its relationship with health and wellbeing: The threshold concept for occupational therapy. *Australian Occupational Therapy Journal, 61*, 293-298.

Frolek Clark, G., & Chandler, B. E. (Eds.). (2013). *Best practices for occupational therapists in schools.* AOTA Press.

Garfinkel, M., & Seruya, F. M. (2018). Therapists' perceptions of the 3:1 service delivery model: A workload approach to school-based practice. *Journal of Occupational Therapy, Schools, and Early Intervention, 11*, 273-290. https://doi.org/10.1080/19411243.2018.1455551

Grajo, L. C., Laverdure, P., Weaver, L. L., & Kingsley, K. (2020). Becoming critical consumers of evidence in occupational therapy for children and youth. *American Journal of Occupational Therapy, 74*(2), 7402170020. https://doi.org/10.5014/ajot.2020.742001

Handley-More, D., Bruegger, T., Costello, P., & Garfinkel, M. (2019, April). Exploring the role of occupational therapy in supporting literacy across the lifespan. Paper presented at the AOTA Annual Conference & Expo, New Orleans, LA.

Handley-More, D., Wall, E., Orentilcher, M. L., & Hollenbeck, J. (2013). Working in early intervention and school settings: Current views of best practice. *Early Intervention & School Special Interest Section Quarterly, 20*(2), 1-4.

Hansen, R. H., & Hinojosa, J. (1999). Occupational therapy's commitment to nondiscrimination and inclusion position paper. *American Journal of Occupational Therapy, 53*(6), 598.

Hasselkus, B. R. (2011). *The meaning of everyday occupation.* SLACK Incorporated.

Hinojosa, J., & Kramer, P. (1997). Statement--fundamental concepts of occupational therapy: Occupation, purposeful activity, and function. *The American Journal of Occupational Therapy, 51*(10), 864-866. https://doi.org/10.5014/ajot.51.10.864

Hinojosa, L., & Kramer, P. (2017) Occupation as a goal. In J. Hinojosa, P. Kramer, & C. Brasic Royeen (Eds.), *Perspectives on human occupation* (pp. 65-91). F. A. Davis Company.

Howell, D. (2009). Occupational therapy students in the process of interprofessional collaborative learning: A grounded theory study. *Journal of Interprofessional Care, 23*(1), 67-80.

Ikiugu, M. (2007). *Psychosocial conceptual practice models in occupational therapy: Building adaptive capability.* Elsevier.

Ikiugu, M. (2012). Use of theoretical conceptual practice models by occupational therapists in the US: A pilot study. *International Journal of Therapy and Rehabilitation, 19*(11), 629-637. https://doi.org/10.12968/ijtr.2012.19.11.629

Ikiugu, M., & Rosso, H. (2003). Facilitating professional identity in occupational therapy students. *Occupational Therapy International, 10*, 206-225. https://doi.org/10.1002/oti.186

Individuals with Disabilities Education Act of 2004, Pub. L. 108-446, 20 U.S.C. §§ 1400-1482 (2004).

Jackson, L. L. (Ed.). (2007). *Occupational Therapy Services for Children and Youth under IDEA* (3rd ed.). American Occupational Therapy Association.

Kaplan, S., & Seruya, F. M. (2019, April). *Evaluation and goal writing practices of school-based occupational therapists* (Unpublished doctoral thesis). Quinnipiac University, Hamden, CT.

Kielhofner, G. (2009). *Conceptual foundations of occupational therapy practice.* F. A. Davis Company.

Laverdure, P. (2018). Collecting participation-focused evaluation data across the school environment. *Special Interest Section Quarterly Practice Connections, 3*(20), 5-7.

Laverdure, P., Cosbey, J., Gaylord, H., & LeCompte, B. (2017). Providing contextual and collaborative service in school contexts and environments. *OT Practice, 22*(15), CE-1-CE-8.

Laverdure, P., & Rose, D. (2012). Educational relevance in school-based occupational and physical therapy. *Physical & Occupational Therapy in Pediatrics, 32*, 347-354.

Laverdure, P., Stephenson, P., & McDonald, M. (2019). Using the occupational therapy practice framework to guide the evaluation process and make assessment choices in school practice. *OT Practice, 24*(2), CE1-CE8.

Law, M., Steinweinder, S., & Leclair, L. (1998). Occupation, health and well-being. *Canadian Journal of Occupational Therapy, 65*(2), 81-91.

Lee, S. W., Taylor, R., Kielhofner, G., & Fisher, G. (2008). Theory in practice: A national survey of therapists who use the Model of Human Occupation. *American Journal of Occupational Therapy, 62*(1), 106-117. https://doi.org/10.5014/ajot.62.1.106

Lipsky, D. K., & Gartner, A. (2012). *Inclusion: A service not a place.* Dude Publishing.

Muhlenhaupt, M. (2010). The perspective of context as related to frame of reference. In P. Kramer & J. Hinojosa (Eds.), *Frames of reference for pediatric occupational therapy* (pp. 67-95). Lippincott Williams & Wilkins.

Nelson, D. (1996). Therapeutic occupation: A definition. *American Journal of Occupational Therapy, 50,* 775-782. https://doi.org/10.5014/ajot.50.10.775

Nielson, C. (1998). How can the academic culture move toward occupation-centered education? *American Journal of Occupational Therapy, 52*(5), 386-387. https://doi.org/10.5014/ajot.52.5.386

O'Neal, S., Dickerson, A. E., & Holbert, D. (2007). The use of theory by occupational therapists working with adults with developmental disabilities. *Occupational Therapy in Health Care, 21*(4), 71-85. https://doi.org/10.1080/J003v21n04_04

Pierce, D. (2001). Untangling occupation and activity. *American Journal of Occupational Therapy, 55,* 138-146. https://doi.org/10.5014/ajot.55.2.138

Polichino, J. E., & Jackson, L. (2014). Frequently asked questions: Transforming caseload to workload in school-based occupational therapy services. https://www.aota.org/~/media/Corporate/Files/Secure/Practice/Children/Workload-fact.pdf

Reilly, M. (1962). Occupational therapy can be one of the greatest ideas of 20th century medicine (Eleanor Clarke Slagle lecture). *American Journal of Occupational Therapy, 16,* 1-9.

Sadlo, G. (2016). Threshold concepts for educating people about human engagement in occupation: The study of human systems that enable occupation. *Journal of Occupational Science, 23*(4), 496-509.

Schell, B. A., & Schell, J. W. (2008). Professional reasoning as the basis of practice. In B. A. Schell & J. W. Schell (Eds). *Clinical and professional reasoning in occupational therapy.* Wolters Kluwer/Lippincott Williams & Wilkins.

Seruya, F. M., & Ellen, K. M. (2015). Role of the middle school occupational therapist: An initial exploration. *Early Intervention & School Special Interest Section Quarterly, 22*(2), 1-4.

Seruya, F. M., & Garfinkel, M. (2018). Implementing contextually based services: Where do we begin? *SIS Quarterly Practice Connections, 3*(3), 4-6.

Seruya, F. M., & Garfinkel, M. (2020). Caseload and workload: Current trends in school-based practice. *American Journal of Occupational Therapy, 74*(5), 7405205090p1-7405205090p8.

Shogren, K. A., Gross, J. M. S., Forber-Pratt, A. J., Francis, G. L., Satter, A. L., Blue-Banning, M., & Hill, C. (2015). The perspectives of students with and without disabilities on inclusive schools. *Research and Practice for Persons with Severe Disabilities, 40,* 243-260. https://doi.org/10.1177/1540796915583493

Smith, E., & Mackenzie, L. (2011). How occupational therapists are perceived within inpatient mental health settings: The perceptions of seven Australian nurses. *Australian Occupational Therapy Journal, 58*(4), 251-260.

Spencer, K. C., Turkett, A., Vaughan, R., & Koenig, S. (2006). School-based practice patterns: A survey of occupational therapists in Colorado. *American Journal of Occupational Therapy, 60,* 81-91.

U.S. Department of Education. (2007). Laws and guidance: archived: A 25 year history of the IDEA. https://eric.ed.gov/?id=ED556111

Watt, H., & Gage Richards, L. (2016). Factors influencing occupational therapy practitioners' use of push-in and pull-out service delivery models in the school system. *American Journal of Occupational Therapy, 70,* 7011510205p1. https://doi.org/10.5014/ajot.2016.70S1-PO3068

Whiteford, G., & Wilcock, A. (2001). Centralizing occupation in occupational therapy curricula: Imperative of the new millennium. *Occupational Therapy International, 8*(2), 81-85.

Wilcock, A. A., & Townsend, E. (2000). Occupational justice: Occupational terminology interactive dialogue. *Journal of Occupational Science, 7,* 84-86.

Wilcock, A. A., & Townsend, E. A. (2014). Occupational justice. In B. A. B. Schell, G. Gillen, & M. Scaffa (Eds.), *Willard and Spackman's occupational therapy* (12th ed., pp. 541-552). Wolters Kluwer Health/Lippincott Williams & Wilkins.

Wong, S. R., & Fischer, A. (2015). Comparing and using occupation-focused models. *Occupational Therapy in Health Care, 29*(3), 297-315. https://doi.org/10.3109/07380577.2015.1010130

World Health Organization. (2002). *Towards a common language for functioning, disability, and health: ICF – The International Classification of Functioning, Disability and Health.* https://cdn.who.int/media/docs/default-source/classification/icf/icfbeginnersguide.pdf

Yerxa, E. (1998). Occupation: The keystone of a curriculum for a self-defined profession. *American Journal of Occupational Therapy, 52*(5), 265-372.

Zemke, R., & Clark, F. (1997). *Occupational science: The evolving discipline.* F. A. Davis Co.

Theory-Based Decision Making in School Practice

Francine M. Seruya, PhD, OTR/L, FAOTA
and Patricia Laverdure, OTD, OTR/L, BCP, FAOTA

Chapter Objectives

1. Identify the unique considerations of practice in education settings.
2. Describe the way in which occupation, activity, and function are defined and how occupational therapy practitioners address and promote function in the students they serve.
3. Compare and contrast how occupations are highlighted and prioritized in school settings and how they are supported by occupational therapy practitioners.
4. Explore the use of a structured framework to examine data; develop theoretical approaches; and make recommendations with and on behalf of students, teams, schools, and school districts.

Occupational therapy practice in school systems in the United States is framed by shared assumptions of the nature of educationally relevant occupation and the role of engagement in occupations of meaning as a means to health, well-being, and quality of life (American Occupational Therapy Association [AOTA], 2020a). Although there is a dearth of evidence supporting these assumptions (Hammell, 2009; Mocellin, 1995, 1996), when looked at through the lens of the educational setting, clarifying the factors on which a contextually aligned theory, practice model, or frame of reference is situated can provide decision-making guidance across the domains of concern in occupational therapy school practice. The key factors on which such an approach is supported are guided by the fourth edition of the *Occupational Therapy Practice Framework: Domain and Process*

Laverdure, P., & Seruya, F. M. *Theory in School-Based*
Occupational Therapy Practice: A Practical Application (pp. 27-38).
DOI: 10.4324/9781003526773-3

(*OTPF-4*; AOTA, 2020a); the purpose, structure, and function of the U.S. public school system; the roles of occupational therapy as a related service as per the Individuals with Disabilities Education Act (IDEA) of 2004 (AOTA, 2020a); and the emerging body of evidence regarding participation and quality of life for children and youth.

The Charge and Scope of Occupational Therapy in Educational Settings

Like most settings in which occupational therapy practitioners practice, the educational setting offers a unique lens through which decisions are made and practice is implemented. In a setting that is beholden to federal, state, and local educational regulation, policy, and procedure as well as professional guidance and regulation, it is important for practitioners to be cognizant of the charge and scope of service provision. IDEA states that the purpose for the provision of related services such as occupational therapy is to (a) improve, develop, or restore functions impaired or lost through illness, injury, or deprivation; (b) improve the ability to perform tasks for independent functioning if functions are impaired or lost; and (c) prevent, through early intervention, initial or further impairment or loss of function (IDEA, 2004).

The Nature of a Focus on Function

In the IDEA statute, the term *function* appears more than 1200 times, nearly three times that of the frequency of the word academic, and functional performance appears 28 times in the statute. Over its years of revision, although many commenters suggested that the statute include a definition of the word *function*, a definition is not included because "it is a term that is generally understood to refer to skills or activities that are not considered academic or related to a child's academic achievement. Instead, 'functional' is often used in the context of routine activities of everyday living" (U.S. Department of Education, 2006, p. 46661). The commentary provided in the *Federal Register* highlights that in addition to supporting student academic achievement, a student's Individualized Education Program (IEP) must also address their unique and specific functional skills that will be required for them to succeed in academic, living, and work environments after graduation. In this context, functional skills refer to those routine activities of everyday life, such as communication, mobility, activities of daily living (ADLs) and instrumental activities of daily living (IADLs), work, leisure, and social participation, and a statement of the student's functional performance is a mandatory component of each IEP (IDEA, 2004). Section 1414(d)(1)(A)(i)(I) of the act requires that the IEP team document the student's present levels of both academic achievement and functional performance in the plan.

In the context of the educational setting, function may be viewed as the activities that are natural or intended for students to participate. The use of the word *activity* is also notable because it holds specific meaning within the occupational therapy profession. As we discussed in Chapter 2, activity and occupation are often used interchangeably throughout the profession (AOTA, 2020a); yet, many theorists see them as distinct from one another. Some theorists have indicated that activities are those tasks that are part of and make up occupations (Boyt et al., 2014; Hinojosa et al., 2017). Others postulate that activities in and of themselves may be considered occupations (Law et al., 1997;

Wilcock & Townsend, 2014). Regardless of the meaning attributed to the word *activity*, we consider a student's ability to perform activities that are typical and expected within the educational setting to fall within the purview of occupational therapy practice.

Discerning Occupation, Activity, and Function

As noted in Chapter 2, many definitions of occupation can be found in the occupational therapy literature. The ordinary, routine, habitual, taken for granted parts of our daily lives and the special parts of our lives that carry symbolic meaning can both be described as occupations. Human biological needs for sustenance, self-care, shelter, and safety are met through what people do; yet, we know that survival needs alone are insufficient for good health. Humans have a biological need to engage in occupation, and participation in occupation is a biological imperative that is essential to individual and species survival (Wilcock, 1993). Wilcock (1993) suggested that through our evolution, humans have developed the capacity to participate, and the reward of engagement in occupation provides the foundation for an individual's sense of meaning, purpose, satisfaction, fulfillment, and well-being. One's physical, mental, social, emotional, and spiritual health is dependent on participation in occupation. Townsend (1997) argued that occupation is life itself. She suggested that occupations are the active processes of taking care of oneself and others, enjoying life and others in it, and finding satisfying productivity in the contexts in which we function. In their philosophy statement of occupational therapy practice, Hooper and Wood (2019) suggested the following:

> A core philosophical assumption of the profession, therefore, is that by virtue of our biological endowment, people of all ages and abilities require occupation to grow and thrive; in pursuing occupation, humans express the totality of their being, a mind-body-spirit union. Because human existence could not otherwise be, humankind is, in essence, occupational by nature. (p. 46)

The World Federation of Occupational Therapists (WFOT) suggested that occupations are the ways in which individuals, communities, and populations occupy time and bring meaning to their lives (WFOT, 2012). Occupations are the purposeful everyday activities that we need and want to do and that we are expected to do (WFOT, 2012). Occupation is a "specific individual's personally constructed, non-repeatable experience" (Pierce, 2001, p. 139). It is subjective, and it has temporal, spatial, and sociocultural characteristics that are unique to the person engaged at that moment in the specific occupation. Authoring a story about one's experience on a field trip is a unique occupational experience for a student. Although holding a pencil and writing letters, words, and paragraphs on a piece of paper may be universally and conceptually identified and a repeatable and frequent school activity, writing about the field trip experience on that specific day and in that specific context is uniquely understood by the student doing the reflection and writing.

The AOTA, in its summative document describing the inter-related constructs that describe occupational therapy practice (i.e., the *OTPF-4*; AOTA, 2020a), includes the following nine areas of occupation of central interest to occupational therapy practitioners:

1. ADLs may include bathing, showering, toileting, toilet hygiene, grooming, dressing, swallowing, feeding, eating, functional mobility, sexual activity, and personal device care. Additional ADL occupations in the educational setting may include hanging up one's coat in the cubby, placing personal items in a locker, and dressing out for physical education.

2. IADLs may include care of others (childcare), care of pets, community mobility and driving, financial management, meal preparation and cleanup, and safety. Classroom responsibilities such as washing the board, putting away collective materials, and organizing the bookshelf are examples of IADL occupations.

3. Health management may include developing, managing, and maintaining routines for health and wellness. Students in the classroom setting engage in health management occupations as they make choices for snacks, take care of their personal devices (communication, glasses, and mobility devices), notify others when they are not feeling well, and regulate emotional responses to the environment.

4. Rest and sleep may include routines involving rest, sleep preparation, and sleep participation. In the educational settings, students engage in rest and sleep occupations by recognizing the need to relax and rest and engaging in quiet and restful routines in the classroom.

5. Education occupations may include formal and/or informal education participation and interest exploration. Occupational therapy practitioners in educational settings may be engaged in academic, nonacademic, and extracurricular occupations with the students they support.

6. Work occupations may include interest exploration; employment seeking, acquisition, and performance; and volunteer exploration and participation. Students may be involved in work training programs and explore a variety of work occupations as they prepare for transition to postsecondary education and work settings.

7. Play includes play exploration and participation. Students engage in a myriad of play occupations in the school settings to include exploration and pretend play, games (with and without rules), and constructive play. They interact with a variety of play materials and toys throughout their educational experience.

8. Leisure occupations include both leisure exploration and participation. Examining and building skills in leisure pursuits is of common interest to students and school teams. Students often engage in identifying leisure interests, skills, and opportunities as they grow and develop.

9. Social participation includes social interaction with family, peers, friends, and community members. Social participation occupations abound in educational settings as students interact with teachers and teaching staff and other students in the classroom and in other settings (i.e., cafeteria, playground, and hallways).

Among these areas, there are a number of prioritized occupations commonly addressed by school practice. These areas are highlighted in Table 3-1.

Linking one's practice explicitly to occupations of value to students and schools requires knowledge of (a) the occupations themselves, (b) the path to learning them and generalizing them across settings and contexts, and (c) the ways to intervene to support the acquisition of them. Research has shown increasing efficacy and frequency of the use of occupation as an intervention and outcome in practice with children and youth (Kreider et al., 2014), and its use as a means to an end contributes to client and provider satisfaction (Estes & Pierce, 2012; Gray, 1998). The conceptual ideas of occupational therapy, or the profession's theoretical foundations, deepen our commitment to occupation and our understanding of how occupation improves student participation and learning and how to effectively support occupational engagement of students in the school community.

Framing our scope around the conceptual idea that service delivery must be geared to facilitating a student's ability to complete those activities within the school day that are natural and intended allows practitioners to have a philosophical foundation on which they can base their interventions. Conceptually framing the paradigm on which services are provided also allows practitioners to

TABLE 3-1

Areas of Occupation Prioritized in Occupational Therapy Services

AREA OF OCCUPATION	EXAMPLES OF WAYS OCCUPATION IS ADDRESSED IN EDUCATIONAL SERVICE DELIVERY
ADLs	• Managing school arrival and dismissal routines (e.g., transitioning to/from classroom, don/doff outerwear, putting belongings away) • Managing lunch line and cafeteria routines (e.g., transitioning through the lunch line, collecting and paying for food items, transporting tray to table, eating) • Managing personal care and toileting • Dressing out for physical education • Managing health care needs (e.g., medication management, self-catheterization, orthotic wearing schedules) • Managing positioning and mobility and transitioning between places and spaces
IADLs	• Taking care of one's learning space (e.g., desk, locker) • Fulfilling classroom responsibilities and jobs (e.g., line leader, clean the board, serving as a leader of a learning group) • Participating in chores and family routines at home • Participating in community-based outings (e.g., visits to community helpers, grocery store, restaurants)
Health management	• Regulating emotions • Identifying and reporting health-related needs • Making healthy food choices in the classroom and cafeteria • Managing medication routines/schedules • Maintaining personal devices
Rest and sleep	• Regulating the phases of the school day • Supporting sleep hygiene practices at home
Education	• Accessing school materials • Participating in small and large group learning activities (e.g., circle time, table groups, learning centers, group activities) • Participating in independent learning activities (e.g., written language, mathematics, history, science) • Completing schoolwork activities (e.g., seat work, homework) • Participating in creative activities (e.g., art, music)

(continued)

TABLE 3-1 (CONTINUED) **Areas of Occupation Prioritized in Occupational Therapy Services**	
AREA OF OCCUPATION	**EXAMPLES OF WAYS OCCUPATION IS ADDRESSED IN EDUCATIONAL SERVICE DELIVERY**
Work	• Expressing learning (e.g., handwriting, keyboarding, assistive devices, augmentative communication devices) • Managing training, volunteer, and paid work responsibilities (e.g., school building jobs [lost and found cart and school store], community-based volunteer and/or job responsibilities)
Play and leisure	• Exploration of the environment and the materials in it • Identification of interests and making choices • Participating in physical education games and sports • Engaging in recreational activities with classmates (e.g., playground) • Participating in extracurricular activities
Social participation	• Engaging with school mates in learning and recreational activities • Participating as a member of and belonging to the school community

understand certain assumptions related to school-based activity. Based on the definition of function and activity, practitioners must appreciate that these will change over time because what is typical and expected of a child in elementary school will be far different than those of a student in high school. Likewise, the activities may not be student directive. We assert this as an important distinction. Although definitions of occupation and activity are prolific in the use of terms such as *meaningful* and *self-directed*, as school-based practitioners, we are aware of many circumstances in which we provide intervention related to activities in which students may, in fact, place no intrinsic value. An example of this may be completing handwriting tasks for a student who does not enjoy or want to write or facilitating social interaction for a child with limited interest in others. Framing our base on the premise that interventions must be targeted to allow the student to complete those activities that are expected provides affordances for these situations. Finally, practitioners need to consider the sociocultural context in which they are providing services if intervention is to facilitate engagement in typical and intended activities because these will be highly dependent on the social and cultural norms of a particular school or classroom setting.

This conceptual foundation provides a vehicle in which we can determine those areas of focus that are appropriate for intervention within the school setting. Based on a review of the *OTPF-4* (AOTA, 2020a) and relevant literature within school-based practice, there appear to be two broad categories of intervention in which most activities fall:

1. Access: Interventions that provide students the ability to use or interact with academic content and instruction, objects, people, or environments within the school setting.

2. Participation: Interventions that address the students' engagement in interactions and activities.

By focusing on the areas of access and participation, practitioners develop interventions that are designed to address physical space and the objects within it, learning and achievement, and social engagement to allow students to function and engage in student occupations and the occupation of education.

THEORETICAL FOUNDATIONS TO GUIDE DECISION MAKING IN EDUCATIONAL PRACTICE

The roles occupational therapy practitioners fill and their use of theoretical foundations for decision making in school practice vary depending on the needs of the physical and social environment; the personal and cultural context; the student's client factors and performance skills and patterns; and the occupations, roles, and routines that are valued and required by the student and context (AOTA, 2020a). A model that guides occupational therapy practitioners to make clinical decisions and then leads them to choose systematically from an array of theoretical foundations to address the complex and, at times, overlapping or competing challenges impacting occupational participation in schools can be valuable to guide practice in school settings.

Decision making is complex in any setting. In school settings, occupational therapy practitioners are called on to collect data and make decisions collaboratively with the interprofessional team (e.g., the student, caregivers, educators, related services providers). The systematic use of a decision-making schema and the subsequent use of complementary theoretical foundations enable practitioners to consider and evaluate participation impacts and priorities, design effective interventions to support participation, and articulate occupational therapy's distinct contribution and value to interventions developed across each of the domains of concern in occupational therapy school practice (Ikiugu, 2012; Ikiugu & Smallfield, 2011).

The occupational therapy process as outlined in the *OTPF-4* (AOTA, 2020a) provides a tool around which occupational therapy practitioners can engage in structural decision making. The process involves four main steps from evaluation to intervention planning, intervention implementation, and intervention review (progress monitoring or outcome assessment). Figure 3-1 illustrates the occupational therapy process and its process steps and considerations.

Although the *OTPF-4* (AOTA, 2020a) offers practitioners the basic structure of occupational therapy service delivery, there is a lack of description and guidance related to the clinical-reasoning and decision-making processes that practitioners need to integrate theory in practice. In her data-driven decision-making (DDDM) framework, Schaaf (2015) drew on the occupational therapy process and promoted further integration of hypothesis generation and evidence in the clinical-reasoning process and identified ways in which occupational therapy practitioners can use data to guide and measure outcomes. The DDDM framework is made up of a series of pragmatic steps that enable occupational therapy practitioners to "Generat[e] hypotheses that are theoretically driven and that use assessment data to identify the factors affecting participation and identifying and measuring outcomes that are both proximal and distal to participation goals" (Schaaf, 2015, p. 3; Figure 3-2).

Schaaf (2015) suggested that the DDDM framework not only supports hypothesis generation and evidence integration into the clinical-reasoning process, but also the process provides the practitioner a tool to systematically evaluate intervention and provide evidence for practice. Although the DDDM framework empowers practitioners to systematize and structure their clinical reasoning and problem solving, contextualize intervention within occupation, use assessment data more thoroughly, and focus on outcome identification and measurement (Schaaf et al., 2013), the conceptualization of hypothesis generation and the use of explicit theory in education practice remain elusive.

Evaluation
Consultation and Screening
Occupational Profile
Analysis of Occupational Performance

Intervention Planning
Goals
Approach (Theory and Evidence)
Referrals and Coordination

Intervention Implementation
Types of Interventions
Progress Monitoring

Intervention Review
(Re-evaluation)
Outcome Measurement
Continue or Discontinue

Evaluation

Screening or Consultation
- Review client history and referral information

Develop Occupational Profile
- History of participation in occupation (background, context/environment, interests, needs, goals)
- Past level of and perceptions of participation in occupation (satisfaction)
- Past medical, developmental, and therapeutic history and effects of

Analysis of Occupational Performance
- Occupations
- Client Factors
- Performance Skills
- Performance Patterns
- Context and Environments

Evaluation Tools
- Interview
- Observation/Activity Analysis
- Test, Measure, Standardized Assessment

Synthesize Evaluation Data

Intervention Planning

Identify Measurable Client-Centered Goals

Consider Occupational Demands
- Relevance and importance
- Objects used
- Space demands
- Social demands
- Sequencing and timing
- Performance skills
- Required body functions/structures

Establish Therapeutic Approach (based upon theory and evidence)
- Create, promote
- Establish, restore
- Maintain
- Modify
- Prevent

Select Outcomes
- Occupational performance
- Improvement/enhancement
- Prevention
- Health and wellness
- Quality of life
- Participation
- Role competence
- Wellbeing
- Occupational justice

Intervention Implementation

Identify and Implement Types of Intervention
- Therapeutic use of occupations and activities
- Interventions to support occupations
- Education
- Training
- Advocacy
- Self-advocacy
- Group intervention
- Virtual intervention

Determine Dosage
- Duration
- Intensity
- Frequency

Monitor Progress

Intervention Review

Re-evaluate Performance, Participation, and Plan
- Outcome measurement

Modify Plan as Needed

Determine Need for Continuation or Discontinuation of Service

Figure 3-1. The occupational therapy process. (Adapted from American Occupational Therapy Association. [2020a]. Occupational therapy practice framework: Domain and process [4th ed.]. *American Journal of Occupational Therapy, 74*[Suppl. 2], 7412410010p1–7412410010p87. https://doi.org/10.5014/ajot.2020.74S2001)

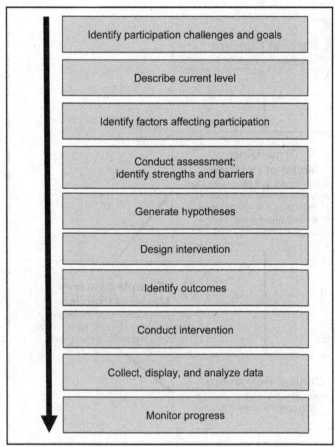

Figure 3-2. The DDDM framework. (Adapted from Schaaf, R. C. [2015]. The issue is: Creating evidence for practice using data-driven decision making. *American Journal of Occupational Therapy, 69,* 6902360010p1-6902360010p6.)

Ikiugu (2007, 2012) developed a systematic decision-making process of choosing theoretical foundations flexibly to address the complexity the of client's needs. The heterogeneous yet systematic process consists of (a) choosing a theoretical model that addresses the client's presenting occupational performance issues, described as the organizing model of practice (OMP), to guide assessment and treatment planning and (b) choosing complementary models of practice (CMPs) that offer compatible assessments and treatment approaches to complement the OMP during evaluation and treatment (Ikiugu, 2007; Ikiugu et al., 2009; Figure 3-3). Ikiugu's (2007) process enables occupational therapy practitioners to systematically combine theoretical foundations that address varying domains of concern and approaches to occupational therapy evaluation and intervention, thereby facilitating the ability to use multiple and theoretically diverse yet compatible approaches.

Considering the reported desire for explicit resources and guidelines to direct school-based practice and the clinical-reasoning process within this distinct setting, the authors have developed a systematic approach to guide practitioners through the occupational therapy process with an

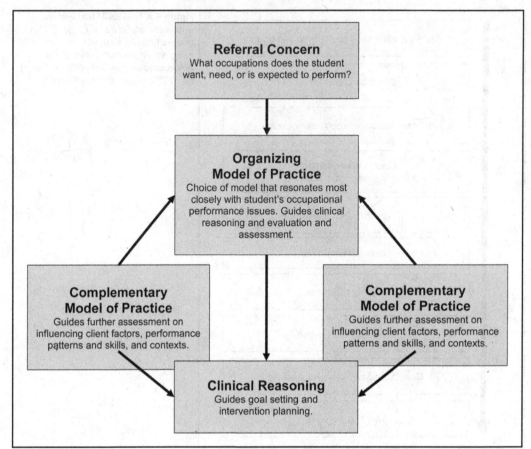

Figure 3-3. Combining theoretical conceptual models. (Adapted from Ikiugu, M. N., Smallfield, S., & Condit, C. [2009]. A framework for combining theoretical conceptual practice models in occupational therapy practice. *Canadian Journal of Occupational Therapy, 76*[3], 162-170. https://doi.org/10.1177/000841740907600305)

emphasis on strong clinical reasoning and theoretical foundation. Using the *OTPF-4*, DDDM, and Ikiugu's process as guiding perspectives, we offer a synthesized and pragmatic approach to guide the use of theory within school-based settings. The following steps are used in the remaining chapters as we discuss salient theoretical frameworks for educational practice:

1. Gather all relevant referral questions and concerns. In educational settings, parental consent is required for any evaluation. Ensure that parental consent has been obtained before proceeding with the evaluation.

2. Complete the occupational profile (AOTA, 2020b) to determine the student's areas of challenges in access or participation. The occupational profile should include information from parents/guardians, teachers, support staff, and the student whenever possible as well as contextually relevant observation of the student and work samples as appropriate.

3. Based on the information gathered in the occupational profile, begin to develop theoretical suppositions regarding rationale for noted challenges.

4. Using theoretical suppositions and determined areas of challenge, conduct initial evaluations. Evaluation processes and standardized and nonstandardized assessment with contextual relevance should align with the theoretical suppositions and identified areas of concern.

5. Identify strengths and challenges to access and participation within the school setting. Determine if and how strengths can be leveraged to mediate barriers.

6.   Collaboratively formulate the desired outcomes and goals to address access and participation.

7.   Based on information gathered through Steps 1 to 5, determine the appropriateness of the initial theoretical suppositions and confirm the OMP of choice.

8.   Consider additional student needs and determine if there are CMPs that are needed to address student-specific challenges and desired student outcomes.

9.   Identify and prioritize goals based on the educational needs, identified priorities, and desired outcomes.

10. Create the intervention plan and implement interventions that align with the OMP and CMPs (e.g., therapeutic use of occupations and activities, interventions to support occupations, education and training, advocacy, group interventions, virtual interventions).

11. Monitor and document student performance and note progress toward the desired outcomes and goals.

CONCLUSION

Occupational therapy practice and decision making in educational settings require the complex integration of factors related to the purpose, structure, and function of the U.S. public school system; the roles of occupational therapy as a related service as outlined by IDEA; the emerging body of evidence regarding participation and quality of life for children and youth; and the professional guidance of the *OTPF-4* (AOTA, 2020a). In school settings, occupational therapy practitioners are called on to collect data across multiple sources and make decisions collaboratively with the inter-professional team (e.g., student, caregivers, educators, related services providers). The systematic use of a decision-making schema and the subsequent use of complementary theoretical foundations enable practitioners to consider and evaluate participation impacts and priorities, design effective interventions to support participation, and articulate occupational therapy's distinct contribution and value to interventions developed across each of the domains of concern in occupational therapy school practice. In the next chapter, we examine the ways in which we use these decision-making schemas to promote collaborative decision making with our school teams.

REFERENCES

American Occupational Therapy Association. (2020a). Occupational therapy practice framework: Domain and process (4th ed.). *American Journal of Occupational Therapy, 74*(Suppl. 2), 7412410010p1-7412410010p87. https://doi.org/10.5014/ajot.2020.74S2001

American Occupational Therapy Association. (2020b). *AOTA occupational profile template.* https://www.aota.org/-/media/Corporate/Files/Practice/Manage/Documentation/AOTA-Occupational-Profile-Template.pdf

Boyt, B., Schell, B., Gillen, G., & Scaffa, M. (Eds.). (2014). *Willard and Spackman's occupational therapy* (12th ed.). Wolters Kluwer Health/Lippincott Williams & Wilkins.

Estes, J., & Pierce, D. (2012). Pediatric therapists' perspectives on occupation-based practice. *Scandinavian Journal of Occupational Therapy, 19*(1), 17-25. https://doi.org/10.3109/11038128.2010.547598

Gray, J. (1998). Putting occupation into practice: Occupation as ends, occupation as means. *American Journal of Occupational Therapy, 52*, 354-364. https://doi.org/10.5014/ajot.52.5.354

Hammell, K. (2009). Sacred texts: A skeptical exploration of the assumptions underpinning theories of occupation. *Canadian Journal of Occupational Therapy, 76*(1), 6-13.

Hinojosa, J., Kramer, P., Royeen, C., & Luebben, A. (2017). In J. Hinojosa, P. Kramer, & C. B. Royeen (Eds.), *Perspectives on human occupation: Theories underlying practice* (pp. 23-37). F. A. Davis.

Hooper, B., & Wood, W. (2019). The philosophy of occupational therapy: A framework for practice. In B. A. B. Schell & G. Gillen (Eds.), *Willard and Spackman's occupational therapy* (13th ed., pp. 43-55). Wolters Kluwer.

Individuals with Disabilities Education Act of 2004, Pub. L. 108-446, 20 U.S.C. § 1400 et seq (2004).

Ikiugu, M. (2007). *Psychosocial conceptual practice models in occupational therapy: Building adaptive capability.* Elsevier.

Ikiugu, M. (2012). Use of theoretical conceptual practice models by occupational therapists in the US: A pilot survey. *International Journal of Therapy and Rehabilitation, 19*(11), 629-637.

Ikiugu, M., & Smallfield, S. (2011). Ikiugu's eclectic method of combining theoretical conceptual practice models in occupational therapy. *Australian Occupational Therapy Journal, 58*(6), 437-446. https://doi.org/10.1111/j.1440-1630.2011.00968.x

Ikiugu, M. N., Smallfield, S., & Condit, C. (2009). A framework for combining theoretical conceptual practice models in occupational therapy practice. *Canadian Journal of Occupational Therapy, 76*(3), 162-170. https://doi.org/10.1177/000841740907600305

Kreider, C. M., Bendixen, R. M., Huang, Y. Y., & Lim, Y. (2014). Review of occupational therapy intervention research in the practice area of children and youth 2009–2013. *American Journal of Occupational Therapy, 68*, e61-e73. https://doi.org/10.5014/ajot.2014.011114

Law, M., Polatajko, H., Baptiste, S., Townsend, E. (1997). Core concepts of occupational therapy. In Canadian Association of Occupational Therapists (Ed.), *Enabling occupation: An occupational therapy perspective* (pp. 29-56). CAOT Publications ACE.

Mocellin, G. (1995). Occupational therapy: A critical overview, part 1. *British Journal of Occupational Therapy, 58*(12), 502-506.

Mocellin, G. (1996). Occupational therapy: A critical overview, part 2. *British Journal of Occupational Therapy, 59*(1), 11-16.

Pierce, D. (2001). Untangling occupation and activity. *American Journal of Occupational Therapy, 55*, 138-146. https://doi.org/10.5014/ajot.55.2.138

Schaaf, R. C. (2015). The issue is: Creating evidence for practice using data-driven decision making. *American Journal of Occupational Therapy, 69*, 6902360010p1-6902360010p6.

Schaaf, R. C., Santalucia, S., & Johnson, C. R. (2013, October). *Creating an evidence based, data-driven model of fieldwork experiences: A collaborative process.* Platform session presented at the American Occupational Therapy Association Education Summit, Atlanta, GA.

Townsend, E. (1997). Inclusiveness: A community dimension of spirituality. *Canadian Journal of Occupational Therapy, 64*(1), 146-155. https://doi.org/10.1177/000841749706400111

U.S. Department of Education. (2006). Assistance to States for the Education of Children With Disabilities and Preschool Grants for Children With Disabilities. Federal Register, 34 CFR Parts 300 and 301. Vol. 71, No. 156. https://www.govinfo.gov/content/pkg/FR-2006-08-14/pdf/06-6656.pdf

Wilcock, A. (1993). A theory of the human need for occupation. *Journal of Occupational Science, 1*(1), 17-24. https://doi.org/10.1080/14427591.1993.9686375

Wilcock, A. A., & Townsend, E. A. (2014). Occupational justice. In B. A. B. Schell, G. Gillen, & M. Scaffa (Eds.), *Willard and Spackman's occupational therapy* (12th ed., pp. 541-552). Wolters Kluwer Health/Lippincott Williams & Wilkins.

World Federation of Occupational Therapists. (2012). *About occupational therapy.* https://www.wfot.org/about-occupational-therapy

Occupation-Based Evaluation

Patricia Laverdure, OTD, OTR/L, BCP, FAOTA
and Francine M. Seruya, PhD, OTR/L, FAOTA

Chapter Objectives

1. Identify the key purposes of evaluation in educational settings.
2. Describe what is meant and the value of an occupation-based evaluation that is designed and conducted from the top down.
3. Explore the attributes of a strength-based, authentic, and collaborative evaluation design grounded in theory to provide a detailed description of the student as an occupational being, their strengths and needs, and a prediction of their educational trajectory.
4. Examine an array of occupation-based assessments to facilitate the collection of data regarding occupational participation and performance.

Occupational therapy practitioners in educational settings use a variety of theoretical approaches to design evaluation and intervention for the clients they serve. Bissell and Cermack (2015) suggested that occupational therapy practitioners use an expanding array of theoretical foundations to include motor learning and sensory integration theories, cognitive and psychosocial models, ecological models, dynamic systems approaches, and occupational-based models such as the Person-Environment-Occupation model or the Person-Environment-Occupation-Performance (PEOP) model. The Person-Environment-Occupation model began to take shape in the late 1980s and early 1990s, at a time in the history of occupational therapy's prolific advancement of its theoretical

Laverdure, P., & Seruya, F. M. *Theory in School-Based Occupational Therapy Practice: A Practical Application* (pp. 39-60). DOI: 10.4324/9781003526773-4

foundations (particularly those that focused on holistic and client-centered approaches), the expansion of ideas around the use of clinical reasoning in the occupational therapy process (Mattingly & Fleming, 1994; Rogers, 1983), and the emergence of occupational science constructs (Yerxa, 1990). Informed by similar ideas, the PEOP model quickly followed, and the two models gave rise to a deeper understanding of occupation as the essential functions that people need and want to do to engage in their daily lives. The expansion of these ideas occurred at the same time that occupational therapy practitioners, rich in theoretical practice underpinnings in mechanistic, reductionistic, and biomedical views of occupational therapy practice, entered educational practice in response to the passage of Public Law 94-142, the Education for All Handicapped Children Act.

Revisions in the public law gradually expanded services and began requiring state and local educational agencies to (a) provide education to students with disabilities in their neighborhood schools; (b) focus that education on the students' participation in curricular activities alongside their nondisabled peers; and (c) consider students' postsecondary outcomes in independent living, education, and vocation. Although during the early history of occupational therapy practice in educational settings, occupational therapy practitioners were demonstrating changes in client factors using these theoretical foundations, they simultaneously found themselves working on the periphery of the students' educational experience. Stages, hallways, and stairwells were common practice settings, and the development of skill acquisition, visual perceptual efficiency, muscle strength, and muscle control was a common goal. Many occupational therapy practitioners soon recognized a need for a paradigm shift in theoretical approaches to effectively meet the needs of students within their challenging educational environments as defined by the Individuals with Disabilities Education Act (IDEA), and occupation-based models such as the PEOP model provided an effective foundation to support this transition. As discussed in Chapter 3, when using occupation-based theoretical foundations to guide our professional reasoning, we not only maximize student outcomes but also most effectively articulate our contributions and distinct value to students, teams, schools, and school districts (Estes & Pierce, 2012). However, in public schools, there is more work to be done in shifting our evaluation and assessment practices from impairment focused to occupation based (Kiraly-Alvarez, 2015).

In public school settings, the purpose of evaluation is to determine the following: (a) Does the student have a disability? (b) Is the disability adversely affecting the student's involvement and progress in general education? and (c) Does the student need specially designed instruction (SDI) as a result of their disability? Therefore, the educational team is responsible for determining the extent to which a student's disability adversely impacts their educational participation and achievement. The team must document whether the disability affects the area of academics (e.g., grades, difficulty with schoolwork) or their functional, social, emotional, and/or behavioral participation or progress. The team must use relevant, multimodal, multicontext, and functional data collected from multiple informants to identify the educational needs of the student and support their determination of needs. If the student is found to be in need of SDI to make academic and functional progress, they are found eligible for special educational services. Occupational therapists offer the team a holistic understanding of student engagement and the affordances and barriers that influence it. Careful discernment through the evaluation process enables the occupational therapist to promote student access to the general curriculum to meet the educational standards that apply to all children and, if found eligible for special education services, resources that support the adaptation of content, methodology, or delivery of instruction to address the unique needs of the student that result from their disability.

ASSESSING PARTICIPATION IN OCCUPATION

The fourth edition of the *Occupational Therapy Practice Framework: Domain and Process* (OTPF-4) describes the three main components to the evaluation of occupational performance and participation as evaluation, planning and delivery of intervention, and the identification and achievement of outcomes (American Occupational Therapy Association [AOTA], 2020a). The purpose of the evaluation is to identify what the client wants and needs to do, what they can do, and what affordances and barriers influence participation and performance.

An occupation-based evaluation is often described as top down because it begins with a focus on the student's occupations, roles, and the ways in which they engage in their daily life. In contrast, diagnostic factors, more commonly addressed initially in a bottom-up approach, focus on deficits and tend to frame performance from a component perspective (i.e., motor control, visual perception, and developmental delay). The occupation-based evaluation designed by the occupational therapist is (a) strength and participation focused; (b) conducted in authentic environments in which students engage (e.g., classroom, playground, cafeteria, art room, music room, after-school settings, community, home); and (c) guided by team collaboration. It provides a description of the student from a contextual lens, gives an understanding of strengths and needs, informs decisions about needs and intervention, and predicts educational trajectory and outcomes.

The first step in the evaluation process is to gather information regarding the client's (student, teacher, or caregiver) perception of the student's, context's, and occupation's impact on occupational performance (Baum et al., 2015). The occupational profile provides an overview of the client's occupational history, their interests and values, their occupational needs, and the contexts in which they participate. Through the occupational profile narrative, data are gathered about the student's (a) history of participation in occupation (background, context/environment, interests, needs, and goals) and how participation may have been influenced by background, context, environment, interests, needs, and goals; (b) subjective experience of participation (strengths and needs) in occupation and how participation is influenced by desire, satisfaction, and performance; and (c) participation expectations and goals (what they need and want to do). At the outset of the evaluation process, the occupational therapist gathers relevant information about the student's participation from a variety of sources including the educational record, the referral request, the teacher and parent, the classroom expectations, and the student. Table 4-1 provides a list of common data collected for the occupational profile.

Understanding the value of occupation in the lives of the student is critical to supporting access and participation. Although a student's participation in occupation can be observed, interpretation of the meaning or emotional content of an occupation by anyone other than the person experiencing it is necessarily inexact (Dickie et al., 2006; Pierce, 2001). In addition, the value of occupation and occupational engagement varies across the developmental trajectory. Table 4-2 illustrates the ways in which expectations and demands influence occupation, contextual, and environmental factors across the age and grade levels as a student progresses through the educational system.

TABLE 4-1

Common Data Collected for the Occupational Profile

What concerns do the student and their team have about the student's occupational engagement?	Describe in what ways the student is struggling to participate in school. • Consider the nine areas of occupation described in Chapter 3.
In what occupations is the student successful, and what barriers impact their success?	Describe the ways that the student is successful and the barriers that impact success.
What is the student's occupational history?	Describe the occupations the student can or does engage in.
What are the student's and team's personal interests and values?	Describe the values and interests of the student, caregivers, and educational staff.
What aspects of the contexts do the student and their team see as supporting engagement in desired occupations, and what aspects are inhibiting engagement? • As with occupations, contexts change as students progress through the life span. Not only are contexts and environments influenced by the individual that is interacting within them, but they change over time given the occupational expectations and demands on students as they grow. For example, as the student develops, the educational environment shifts from the small group setting of preschool to the increasingly large and distant environment of the high school or postsecondary settings.	
ENVIRONMENT	Describe the following: • Physical: Natural and/or built surroundings and the nonhuman elements (animals, plants, tools, materials, and buildings) and objects in them • Social: People, groups, and populations with whom one is in contact and with whom one has a relationship
PERSONAL	Describe the following: • Age, sex, socioeconomic and educational status, and group membership (features that are not part of health condition) • Customs, beliefs, behavior patterns, and expectations accepted by society and from which one draws identity and occupational choices
PERFORMANCE PATTERNS	Describe the following: • Habits: Acquired tendencies to respond in consistent ways in familiar environments or situations; specific behaviors performed repeatedly, automatically, and with little variation • Routines: Patterns of behaviors (promoting or damaging) that are observable, repetitive, embedded in cultural/ecological contexts, and add structure to daily life • Rituals: Symbolic actions (spiritual, cultural, and social) that contribute to identity and reinforce values and beliefs • Roles: Sets of behaviors that are defined and expected by society and shaped by context and culture

(continued)

TABLE 4-1 (CONTINUED)

Common Data Collected for the Occupational Profile

What client factors do the student and their team see as supporting engagement in desired occupations, and what aspects are inhibiting engagement?

- Client factors are influenced by biological, psychosocial, environmental, and contextual factors and change as students grow and develop. Students experience physical and psychological maturation, which changes their interests and the occupations they participate in. Similarly, the routines and roles they participate in are shaped by the contexts and environments in which they participate. This transactional process not only supports engagement but also influences the developmental trajectory and is described in this section of the occupational profile.

VALUES, BELIEFS, AND SPIRITUALITY	Define the following: • Values: The individual's beliefs and commitment about what is good, right, and important acquired from their cultural experience (Kielhofner, 2008) • Beliefs: The individual's ideas that are held as truths • Spirituality: The ways in which the client seeks and expresses meaning and purpose; their connectedness to the moment, self, others, nature, and the sacred (Puchalski et al., 2009)
BODY FUNCTIONS	Describe the physiological functions of body systems including the following: • Mental functions • Sensory functions (visual, vestibular, hearing, taste, smell, proprioceptive, touch, and pain) • Motor functions (motor reflexes, reactions, and tone) • Movement functions (musculoskeletal, joint stability/mobility, and gait) • Cardiovascular, metabolic hematological, skin, immunological, respiratory, digestive, and reproductive functions • Voice and speech functions
BODY STRUCTURES	Describe the following body structures: • Anatomical parts of the body such as head, limbs, and organs that support function

(continued)

TABLE 4-1 (CONTINUED) **Common Data Collected for the Occupational Profile**	
What are the student's and their team's priorities and desired goals?	
OCCUPATIONAL PERFORMANCE	Occupational performance is the "doing of meaningful activities, tasks, roles through complex interactions between the person and the environment" (Baum et al., 2015, p. 52). Occupational performance is described as an experimental process, not unlike the nature of childhood development, and Baptiste (2017) argues that "to achieve occupational performance, there needs to be a well-coordinated appraisal of the key domains (i.e., person, environment, occupation)" (p. 146). Describe the following: • Motor skills (e.g., aligns, stabilizes, positions, reaches, bends, grips, manipulates, coordinates, moves, lifts, walks, transports, calibrates, flows, endures, paces) • Process skills (e.g., paces, attends, heeds, chooses, uses, inquires, initiates, continues, sequences, terminates, searches/locates, gathers, organizes, restores, navigates, notices/responds, adjusts, accommodates, benefits) • Social interaction skills (e.g., approaches/starts, concludes/disengages, produces speech, gesticulates, speaks fluently, turns toward, looks, places self, touches, regulates, questions, replies, discloses, expresses emotion, disagrees, thanks, transitions, times response, times duration, takes turns, matches language, clarifies, acknowledges and encourages, empathizes, heeds, accommodates, benefits)
PREVENTION	Describe the contextual, performance, and client factor affordances and resiliencies that prevent primary and secondary impairment resulting from limitations in occupational access, participation, and performance.
HEALTH AND WELLNESS	Describe the factors that influence the student's health and wellness.
QUALITY OF LIFE AND WELL-BEING	Describe the factors that influence the student's quality of life and well-being.
PARTICIPATION AND ROLE COMPETENCE	Describe the student's occupational participation and the performance patterns and skills that may influence participation and the student's perception of role competence.
OCCUPATIONAL JUSTICE	Describe the contextual, performance, and client factors that influence the student's ability to engage equally and fairly in expected (e.g., age and grade expectations), meaningful, and healthy occupations.

Adapted from American Occupational Therapy Association. (2020b). AOTA occupational profile template. https://www.aota.org/-/media/Corporate/Files/Practice/Manage/Documentation/AOTA-Occupational-Profile-Template.pdf

TABLE 4-2

Key Occupation, Contextual, and Environmental Influences Across Educational Experience

EDUCATIONAL PLACEMENT	AGE (YEARS)	GRADE	KEY OCCUPATION FACTORS	KEY CONTEXTUAL AND ENVIRONMENTAL FACTORS
Early childhood/ preschool	2 to 5	EC/PS	School self-care routines Social interaction with larger community (classroom)	School transportation (car and bus) Longer school day Safety procedures in the classroom Before- and after-school care
Early elementary	5 to 6	K	Increased developmental and academic demands	Longer school day (kindergarten may be half or full day with transition to full day in first grade) Cafeteria (as well as adjustment to school foods) Safety in the classroom and school building Before- and after-school care
	6 to 7	1	Increased responsibility for self Adjustment in sleep routines	
	7 to 8	2		
Late elementary	8 to 9	3	Increased academic demands Increased self-care/social demands	After-school activities Safety in the classroom, school building, and community Before- and after-school care for some children Increased individualized interests (after-school activities)
	9 to 10	4	Increased responsibilities for the social community (school jobs)	
	10 to 11	5	Increased opportunity for leadership	
	11 to 12	6	Learning challenges Physical growth impact Standardized testing Adjustment to sleep schedule	

(continued)

TABLE 4-2 (CONTINUED)

Key Occupation, Contextual, and Environmental Influences Across Educational Experience

EDUCATIONAL PLACEMENT	AGE (YEARS)	GRADE	KEY OCCUPATION FACTORS	KEY CONTEXTUAL AND ENVIRONMENTAL FACTORS
Middle school	12 to 13	7	Larger student population	Longer school distances
	13 to 14	8	Increased academic demands	Safety in the classroom, school building, and larger community (bullying and other social challenges)
			Choice of academics	
			Social emotional regulation requirements	
			Adjustment to sleep schedule	
High school	14 to 15	9	Increased autonomy	Longer school distances
	15 to 16	10	Adjustment to sleep schedule	Safety and autonomy in the school building and larger community
	16 to 17	11		
	17 to 18	12		

EC/PS, early childhood/preschool; K, kindergarten.

Access and Participation

Occupational therapy practitioners leverage the relationship between the student and the ways in which they value and engage in occupation to promote congruence between their needs and their capacities (Baum et al., 2015). When congruence is optimized, occupational performance is also optimized. In educational settings, occupation-based evaluation provides occupational therapy practitioners with many entry points for evaluation, assessment, and intervention. Using a top-down approach enables occupational therapy practitioners the opportunity to identify and prioritize what is important to the student, caregivers, and teachers and to determine the strengths and challenges that influence access and participation in these meaningful occupations. For example, addressing access features on computers used for writing tasks with children with reading and writing impairments has been shown to significantly improve student engagement, achievement, and satisfaction in written expression. Additionally, creating accessible spaces on the playground significantly improves social participation and perceptions of belonging in children with physical disabilities.

Therefore, one might ask the following question: What are the occupations of interest to occupational therapy practitioners in educational practice? Do we address each and every occupation defined in the *OTPF-4*? Are the occupations nuanced uniquely or weighted differently for practice in the educational setting? As we asserted in Chapter 3, framing our attention to the access and participation challenge that can be organized under an educational vs. a medical paradigm may not prove to be a useful approach. Occupation-based evaluation can free us from the constraints that the educational vs. a medical model limits us to. Examining occupation and the transactional relationships between it, the student, and the factors that influence it requires that we consider all of the factors associated with the student, the context, and the occupation regardless of if those factors are defined in some arbitrary way by a medical condition. Occupational therapy practitioners are uniquely poised to translate knowledge about the factors associated with access and participation in school environments and occupations and to facilitate participation in these environments and occupations in ways that promote achievement in education, health, and wellness outcomes regardless of the medical origin of the influencing factors.

Occupational therapists concern themselves with student access and participation across the student's school day experience. Accessing and managing school transportation to and from school; transitions (ambulating, using a wheelchair, and maintaining secure positions) into, out of, and within the school building and its many instructional and recreational spaces (hallways, classroom, art and music rooms, gym, playground, and after-school settings); managing self-care needs in the classroom, the bathrooms, and the cafeteria (toileting, donning and doffing outerwear, eating, and dressing for physical education); accessing and managing instruction and instructional materials in the classroom for both learning input (accessible learning materials and universal instructional design and implementation) and output (handwriting and assistive technology); and participating in the social community of the classroom and the school are some of the many participatory expectations of our students (Bundy, 1995; Swinth et al., 2007). Occupational therapy practitioners attend to the school life factors that define the roles and routines expected of students in school, and although participation in some of the occupations that comprise these roles and routines may not be identified as valued and meaningful by the student, we recognize its value to the contribution of skill mastery, role identity, and performance competence fundamental for successful postsecondary outcomes (Rodger & Ziviani, 2006).

School life demands as well as childhood developmental trajectories change over the course of a student's experience in their educational journey. Not only is it important to consider the transactional relationship between the student, the school environment, and the school occupations, but it is also critical that the analysis of the congruence among these factors be considered from the context of the student's age and developmental demands and expectations. Table 4-3 illustrates the ways in which the developmental trajectory influences occupational performance in motor, process, and social interaction demands across the childhood life span.

TABLE 4-3

Occupational Performance Demand in Motor, Social Participation, and Process Demand Across the Childhood Life Span

GRADE LEVEL	EDUCATIONAL MOTOR DEMANDS	EDUCATIONAL SOCIAL PARTICIPATION DEMANDS	EDUCATIONAL PROCESS DEMANDS
Early elementary	Eye-hand coordination, stabilization, and praxis Gross motor efficacy	Expanding vocabulary, both general and academic specific Phonological awareness (phoneme memory and manipulation) Speech intelligibility Morphological awareness Beginning reading	Visual discrimination and visual motor integration Trial and error learning
Late elementary	Motor memory and visual motor accuracy Planning simple motor sequences First comparisons of athletic capacity	Specialized educational vocabulary, increasingly through print Use of syntax and morphemes to determine meaning Learning through reading, both informational and fiction Explain knowledge orally and in writing Adapt communication for the audience Use of language to think about language (metalinguistics)	Motor persistence and task completion Spatial and sequential planning Experiential learning

(continued)

TABLE 4-3 (CONTINUED)

Occupational Performance Demand in Motor, Social Participation, and Process Demand Across the Childhood Life Span

GRADE LEVEL	EDUCATIONAL MOTOR DEMANDS	EDUCATIONAL SOCIAL PARTICIPATION DEMANDS	EDUCATIONAL PROCESS DEMANDS
Middle school	Convergence of body image and motor capacities Graphomotor fluency and automaticity Gross motor anticipatory planning	Expansion of informational and narrative reading comprehension skills Adapt written communication for the audience Expository comprehension and expression Use of abstract and figurative language	Extended mental and motor effort and rapid motor responsivity Material management and organization Critical thinking with manual problem-solving (procedural) learning
High school	Graphomotor fluency and automaticity Gross motor specialization	Create a persuasive argument both orally and in writing Research information and integrate into oral and written communication	Production meta-analysis (previewing, pacing, self-monitoring) Process-oriented reasoning/production Synthesis of knowledge from experience

Using a top-down approach, occupational therapy practitioners endeavor to look beyond the client factors that limit access and participation in expected occupation, roles, and routines and address needed changes in occupational opportunities, instructional approaches and materials, and environmental and contextual barriers. This shift from bottom-up approaches that may be considered traditional and desired in some schools may require reframing of teacher's, parent's, and administrator's expectations (Hanft & Shepherd, 2016). Taking the time to build the collaborative relationships; expand the capacity in caregivers, teachers, and administrators; and develop innovative teaching and learning supports, strategies, and technologies required for effective practice significantly changes a student's prospects for authentic participation and belonging in the classroom and school community (Bayona et al., 2006; Case-Smith & Rogers, 2005; Reid et al., 2006; Wehrmann et al., 2006).

EVALUATION AND ASSESSMENT

Educational legislation does not require discipline-specific evaluations (e.g., occupational therapy) as long as the student is evaluated by a qualified professional in all areas of the suspected disability and delineates that the purpose of evaluation in schools is to (a) determine a student's eligibility for special education, (b) gather data for individualized programming planning, and (c) reevaluate for progress monitoring and reporting. We do not assess to determine if the student qualifies for therapy services; instead, we develop and use a variety of evaluation strategies that help the team determine what a student needs in order to receive a free appropriate public education in the least restrictive environment.

An occupation-based evaluation top-down approach aligns structurally and functionally with the occupational therapy evaluation process outlined in the *OTPF-4* (AOTA, 2020a). Top-down evaluation approaches help teams make decisions about the student's ability to participate and perform in the school setting and identify the ways performance challenges affect participation in school activities. Top-down evaluation and decision making focus on (a) establishing the roles that an individual needs or desires to perform, (b) determining the skills required to perform those roles, (c) identifying the resources needed to accomplish those skills, and (d) specifying the remedial and modifying processes that will bring about success. Using this approach, the occupational therapist may ask questions such as (a) Who is the student? (b) What do referrers and the student think is interfering with the learning process and the student's participation? (c) How does the student's engagement and participation compare to peers in the same instructional setting? (d) What are the student's, teacher's, and family's concerns relative to engaging in occupations and daily life activities? and (e) What are the student's, classroom's, and family's areas of strength?

After gathering information about the student's history of participation in occupation, their subjective experience of participation (strengths and needs) in occupation, and their participation expectations and goals, the occupational therapist considers the factors associated with the student, context, and occupation that positively influence or constrain occupational performance. As discussed in Chapter 3, as data are gathered, the occupational therapist begins to form an organizing occupation-based conceptual framework to understand the student's occupational profile (Ikiugu, 2007). In this phase of the evaluation process, the occupational therapist considers the transactional influences of the client factors, the areas of occupation, and the context to identify an organizing conceptual model that frames areas of strength and need and the role that each of these key domains of function plays on occupational performance (Ikiugu & Smallfield, 2015). Observing student participation across environments such as the classroom, playground, and cafeteria and traversing within and between these environments provide an overview of their capacity and participation, the scaffolds needed for successful participation, and the barriers that prevent successful engagement in natural and authentic academic and social contexts. In addition, authentic observation provides validation to our developing theoretical impressions and formulations.

Assessment

Educational legislative mandates require school personnel to use "... assessment tools and strategies that provide *relevant* information that directly assists ... in determining the educational needs of the child ..." (IDEA, 2004). Educational legislation shapes our evaluation processes by requiring that evaluations be (a) selected and administered to avoid discrimination on racial or cultural basis, (b) administered in the child's native language or other mode of communication validated for the specific purpose for which they are used, (c) administered by trained and knowledgeable personnel in accordance with any instructions provided, (d) conducted under standard conditions (or if not, a description of the extent to which it varied from standard conditions must be indicated), and (e) accurately reflective of the individual's aptitude or achievement level or whatever other factors the test purports to measure.

Occupation-based evaluation approaches uniquely equip occupational therapy practitioners to identify the educational needs of students; describe the influence of supports and barriers on participation in meaningful occupation; and prioritize participation based on the student's, family's, and teacher's desired outcomes (AOTA, 2008). Coster (1998) suggested using Trombly's (1993) top-down approaches "as a starting point for building a pediatric assessment guide to the process of information gathering ... that support an occupation-centered assessment process" (p. 339). Coster (1998) posited the following:

> An alternative approach to defining the most global level of assessment concern is to focus on the child's overall pattern of occupational engagement in relation to a particular context of importance ... What matters most is not individual abilities and disabilities with regard to particular tasks, but the extent to which the person is able to construct a pattern of occupational engagement that meets individual needs and goals as well as societal expectations. [Occupational therapists focus on] uncovering the obstacles impeding successful occupational engagement. (pp. 339-340)

Therefore, we assert that assessment using theory and occupation-based approaches begins with an analysis of occupation, and occupation-based assessment tools can be helpful in validating the organizing conceptual model chosen and point to the need for additional complementary models to be used for evaluation and intervention planning. Table 4-4 provides a summary of the available tests and measures to assess the influence of affordances and barriers on occupational participation and performance in the educational setting.

Occupational therapists bring a unique lens of access and meaningful participation to evaluating students in school settings (AOTA, 2014), and other important assessment options for the occupational therapist include the array of tools that evaluate the student's access to and participation within the educational setting. As noted, the core purpose of assessment in educational settings is to determine whether a student has a disability; whether that disability adversely affects the student's participation, performance, and progress in the general education curriculum; and whether the student requires SDI to access and make progress in their educational program (Jackson, 2007). Integrating occupational performance and participation data with the occupational profile in this occupation-based and participation-focused assessment process enables a very thorough holistic analysis of the student's valued occupations and real-life participation, the life roles they fulfill satisfactorily, and what needs they have to succeed.

TABLE 4-4

Tests and Measures to Assess Occupational Performance and Participation

MEASURE	PURPOSE	CONSTRUCTS	AGE	TIME TO ADMINISTER	FORMAT/TYPE OF ADMINISTRATION	FORMAT AND SCORES
Canadian Occupational Performance Measure	Identifies occupational performance problems, defines priorities, and guides goal setting	Measures clients perceived occupational performance in three areas: Self-care, productivity, and leisure	Any age, with or without disabilities	15 to 30 minutes	Semistructured interview by therapist	Standardized scores, norm referenced
Child Occupational Self-Assessment	Captures children and youths' perception regarding sense of occupational competence and importance of everyday activities	How competent does a child feel engaging in and completing activities	8 to 13 years (must have self-reflection and planning skills)	25 minutes	Self-report, structured interview	Importance rating scale, priorities for change
Children's Assessment of Participation and Enjoyment	Examines participation in everyday activities outside of school classes	Multiple dimensions of participation including diversity of activity, frequency, enjoyment, and context	Children with and without disabilities, 6 to 21 years	30 to 45 minutes	Questionnaire, self-report, or interview	Mean intensity and subjective enjoyment

(continued)

TABLE 4-4 (CONTINUED)

Tests and Measures to Assess Occupational Performance and Participation

MEASURE	PURPOSE	CONSTRUCTS	AGE	TIME TO ADMINISTER	FORMAT/TYPE OF ADMINISTRATION	FORMAT AND SCORES
Children's Kitchen Task Assessment	Examines executive function through a task of making playdough	Measures initiation, sequencing, safety judgment, organization, working memory	8 to 12 years	20 minutes	Free downloadable assessment materials	Nonstandardized assessment in which the score is based on the number and type of cues needed to complete the activity. Each step of the activity is scored on a scale of 0 to 5 with 0 = no cues, 1 = general verbal guidance, 2 = gesture guidance, 3 = direct verbal assistance, 4 = physical assistance, and 5 = completing the task for the participant.
Goal-Oriented Assessment of Lifeskills	Assesses functional motor skills required for daily living skills	Measures seven tasks requiring fine or gross motor skills: Utensils, locks, paper box, notebook, carry tray, ball play, and manage clothing	7 to 17 years, with or without disabilities	45 to 60 minutes	Series of seven occupation-based activities	Standard scores, with option to document progress over time

(continued)

TABLE 4-4 (CONTINUED)

Tests and Measures to Assess Occupational Performance and Participation

MEASURE	PURPOSE	CONSTRUCTS	AGE	TIME TO ADMINISTER	FORMAT/TYPE OF ADMINISTRATION	FORMAT AND SCORES
Miller Function and Participation Scales	Assess a child's performance related to school participation with a focus on motor skill performance	Measures mild to moderate delays in visual, fine, and gross motor skills	2.6 to 7.11 years	20 to 30 minutes per subset, 45 to 60 minutes for entire assessment	Workbook/task format, administered by therapist	Standard scores, percentile ranks, age equivalents, and progress scores
Participation and Environment Measure for Children and Youth	Assess participation in the home, at school, and in the community as well as environmental factors of participation	Home, school, and community	5 to 17 years old, with or without disabilities	25 to 40 minutes	Parent report questionnaire	Rating scale of participation frequency, involvement and desire for change and environmental support
Preferences for Activities of Children	Recreational, active physical, social, skill based, and self-improvement	Measures activity preference	6 to 21 years, with or without disabilities	15 to 20 minutes	Self-report or interview	Preferences for involvement in meaningful activities
Pediatric Evaluation of Disability Inventory	Comprehensive assessment of functional skill development and level of independent performance of functional activities in a child's environment	Evaluates capability and performance of functional activities in the domains of self-care, mobility, and social function	0 months to 8 years, physical or combined physical and cognitive disabilities	45 to 60 minutes for administration and scoring	Questionnaire format, administered by parent report, professional judgment, or combination	Standard and scaled performance scores

(continued)

TABLE 4-4 (CONTINUED)

Tests and Measures to Assess Occupational Performance and Participation

MEASURE	PURPOSE	CONSTRUCTS	AGE	TIME TO ADMINISTER	FORMAT/TYPE OF ADMINISTRATION	FORMAT AND SCORES
School Function Assessment	Assessment of functional capabilities and performance of functional activities that support participation in academic and related social aspects of an education program	Participation, task supports, activity performance	5 to 12 years	60 to 90 minutes	Judgment-based questionnaire, interview, or observation	Raw scores, criterion scores 0 to 100 for full grade functioning
Short Child Occupational Profile	Assessment of a child's occupational participation	Measures the influence of volition, habituation, skills, and the environment on participation	Birth to 21 years	20 minutes for administration and scoring	Observational assessment across five sections (volition, habituation, communication and interaction, process skills, and motor skills)	Letter rating scores include F = Facilitates, A = Allows, I = Inhibits, and R = Restricts.

Adapted from Laverdure, P., Stephenson, P., & McDonald, M. (2019). Using the occupational therapy practice framework to guide the evaluation process and make assessment choices in school practice. *OT Practice, 24*(2), CE1-CE8.

Another advantage to a top-down and theory-guided approach to evaluation is that it allows occupational therapists to identify what a student is capable of doing in a standardized controlled environment, what they can do in their daily environment, and what they actually do in their daily environment (Holsbeeke et al., 2009; Smits-Engelsman et al., 2013). Occupational therapists contribute to the discernment about disability presence and impact by offering valuable information about how responsive a student is to support, modification, and resources and whether or not skills can generalize from one context to another functionally.

The RIOT (Review, Interview, Observe, Test)/ICEL (Instruction, Curriculum, Environment, Learner) matrix is a framework used by many schools to increase schools' confidence in the quality of the data collected and the findings that emerge from the data (Hosp, 2006, 2008). The RIOT draws from a range of data to consider the possible explanations of academic and functional challenges, confirm/rule out competing explanations, and reduce bias in evaluation and includes the following:

- Review: Consider the student's academic and medical record, concerns expressed by the referral source, curricular demands, and strategies implemented.
- Interview: Discuss strengths and needs with the student, teacher and school staff, and caregivers.
- Observe: Observe the student across a wide variety of environments while engaged in an array of naturally occurring activities.
- Test: Consider the array of tests, measures, and assessments.

The ICEL draws from a range of data to consider the possible influences on student learning as follows:

- Instruction: Consider the instructional methodology and strategies (instruction, modifications, and accommodations).
- Curriculum: What is the impact of curricular demands and expectations?
- Environment: Consider the environmental barriers that impact participation in desired and expected activities.
- Learner: Use of the *OTPF-4* (AOTA, 2020a) to support a thorough understanding of the learner.

Table 4-5 illustrates the way in which the RIOT/ICEL matrix can support the development of a theoretical and top-down approach to the evaluation.

After the occupational profile is established and occupational performance data are collected, in a theory-guided evaluation, the occupational therapist considers the following:

- What patterns and themes emerge in the results?
- Are there any deviations from these patterns? If yes, are there any factors that might explain these deviations?
- Do the results make sense?
- Are the results significant from an academic or functional standpoint?

We may find that at this point our theoretical approach, the occupational profile, and our occupational performance assessment provide sufficient information to support team decision making. At the same time, performance gaps may have been uncovered in the evaluation process that require additional investigation. As these gaps are identified, the occupational therapist develops complementary theoretical assumptions and frames of reference to guide further assessment, identify and explain the challenges, and inform intervention approaches. At times, additional information is required to understand challenges related to client and personal factors and performance skills and patterns (AOTA, 2020a). Assessments used to gather additional information about these factors may include the following:

- School Assessment of Motor and Performance Skills
- Assessment of Life Habits for Children
- Bruininks-Oseretsky Test of Motor Proficiency
- Developmental Test of Visual-Motor Integration

TABLE 4-5

Using the Review, Interview, Observe, Test/Instruction, Curriculum, Environment, Learner Matrix to Guide Evaluation and Theoretical Approach

	REVIEW	INTERVIEW	OBSERVE	TEST
INSTRUCTION	What factors contribute to how the student has performed in school, home, and community?	When is the student able to work independently and successfully?	What strategies are used to support success in participation?	What would the student do to demonstrate their knowledge or skills?
CURRICULUM	What expectations are there of the students in the class?	Where does the student do well academically?	What accommodations and modifications are used to support participation?	What hypotheses have emerged from the data that explain the student's challenges?
ENVIRONMENT	What supports and barriers (physical, sensory, instructional, and social) exist?	What obstacles has the student overcome and what remains challenging?	What resources best support the student's engagement and achievement?	What kinds of things might be helpful to improve the student's access and participation?
LEARNER	In what activities, roles, and routines does the student engage?	What is the student's favorite part of the school day? What does the student enjoy doing at school/home?	In what environments does the student function at their best?	What helps the student be the best that they can be? What does the student need to be able to be their best?

- Developmental Test of Visual Perception
- Evaluation of Social Interaction
- Gross Motor Function Measure
- Manual Ability Classification System
- Pediatric Volitional Questionnaire
- Peabody Developmental Motor Scales
- Sensory Profile
- Sensory Processing Measure
- School Setting Interview

As we conclude our data gathering and analysis, we identify when, why, where, and what factors result in difficulty or prevent a student from performing occupations within their desired roles. We understand the student's interests, motivations, and needs and the biopsychosocial scaffolds that support engagement and the barriers that impede participation in the student's daily occupations and routines. We can share knowledge about the contexts and environments in which the student functions most adaptively and why. Our evaluative information can support the team's discernment of determining eligibility for special education services and/or for the development of an appropriate instructional program that builds skills for employment and independent living beyond school.

Conclusion

Designing an evaluation from the top down and centering it on the occupations that a student values, wants, and needs to do to be an active participant in the classroom, school, and curriculum promotes the overarching purpose of evaluation according to IDEA. By integrating the AOTA's *OTPF-4* (AOTA, 2020a) and the provision of IDEA, we ensure that we gather relevant data that will inform the team's determination of need and eligibility of special education services and the development of effective instructional and intervention approaches. Central to the occupational therapy evaluation, of course, is occupation, and using occupation-based theoretical foundations in the design and implementation of evaluation and assessment in school practice is paramount. As explored in the coming chapters, using occupation-based theoretical foundations will enable a practice that focuses on students' strengths and interests; addresses school participation and performance requirements; and maximizes long-term independent living, postsecondary education, and vocational outcomes.

References

American Occupational Therapy Association. (2008). Occupational therapy practice framework: Domain and process (2nd ed.). *American Journal of Occupational Therapy, 62,* 625-683.

American Occupational Therapy Association. (2014). Occupational therapy practice framework: Domain and process (3rd Ed.). *American Journal of Occupational Therapy, 68*(Supplement_1), S1-S48. https://doi.org/10.5014/ajot.2014.682006

American Occupational Therapy Association. (2020a). Occupational therapy practice framework: Domain and process (4th ed.). *American Journal of Occupational Therapy, 74*(Suppl. 2), 7412410010p1-7412410010p87. https://doi.org/10.5014/ajot.2020.74S2001

American Occupational Therapy Association. (2020b). *AOTA occupational profile template.* https://www.aota.org/-/media/Corporate/Files/Practice/Manage/Documentation/AOTA-Occupational-Profile-Template.pdf

Baptiste, S. (2017). The Person-Environment-Occupation model. In J. Hinojosa, P. Kramer, & C. B. Royeen (Eds.), *Perspectives on human occupation* (pp. 137-159). F. A. Davis.

Baum, C., Christiansen, C., & Bass, J. (2015). The Person-Environment-Occupation-Performance model. In C. Baum, C. Christiansen, & J. Bass (Eds.), *Occupational therapy: Performance, participation, and well-being* (4th ed., pp. 49-56). SLACK Incorporated.

Bayona, C. L., McDougall, J., Tucker, M. A., Nichols, M., & Mandich, A. (2006). School-based occupational therapy for children with fine motor difficulties: Evaluating functional outcomes and fidelity of services. *Physical and Occupational Therapy in Pediatrics, 26*(3), 89-110.

Bissell, J., & Cermack, S. (2015). Frameworks, models, and trends in school-based occupational therapy in the United States. *The Israeli Journal of Occupational Therapy, 24*(2-30), E49-E69.

Bundy, A. C. (1995). Assessment and intervention in school-based practice: Answering questions and minimizing discrepancies. *Physical & Occupational Therapy in Pediatrics, 15,* 69-88.

Case-Smith, J., & Rogers, J. (2005). School-based occupational therapy. In J. Case-Smith (Ed.), *Occupational therapy for children* (5th ed., pp. 795-824). Elsevier Mosby.

Coster, W. (1998). Occupation-centered assessment of children. *American Journal of Occupational Therapy, 52*(5), 337-344. https://doi.org/10.5014/ajot.52.5.337

Dickie, V., Cutchin, M., & Humphry, R. (2006). Occupation as transactional experience: A critique of individualism in occupational science. *Journal of Occupational Science, 13*(1), 83-93. https://doi.org/10.1080/14427 591.2006.9686573

Estes, J., & Pierce, D. (2012). Pediatric therapists' perspectives on occupation based practice. *Scandinavian Journal of Occupational Therapy, 19,* 17-25.

Hanft, B., & Shepherd, J. (2016). *Collaborating for student success: A guide for school-based occupational therapy* (2nd ed.). AOTA Press.

Holsbeeke, L., Ketelaar, M., Schoemaker, M. M., & Gorter, J. W. (2009). Capacity, capability, and performance: Different constructs or three of a kind? *Archives of Physical Medicine and Rehabilitation, 90*(5), 849-855. https://doi.org/10.1016/j.apmr.2008.11.015

Hosp, J. L. (2006). Implementing RTI: Assessment practices and response to intervention. *NASP Communiqué, 34*(7). http://www.nasponline.org/publications/cq/cq347rti.aspx

Hosp, J. L. (2008). Best practices in aligning academic assessment with instruction. In A. Thomas & J. Grimes (Eds.), *Best practices in school psychology V* (pp. 363-376). National Association of School Psychologists.

Ikiugu, M. (2007). *Psychosocial conceptual practice models in occupational therapy: Building adaptive capability.* Elsevier.

Ikiugu, M., & Smallfield, S. (2015). Instructing occupational therapy students in use of theory to guide practice. *Occupational Therapy in Health Care, 29*(2), 165-177. https://doi.org/10.3109/07380577.2015.1017787

Individuals with Disabilities Education Act (IDEA) of 2004, Pub. L. No. 108-446, § 118 Stat. 2647 (2004).

Jackson, L. L. (Ed). (2007). *Occupational therapy services for children and youth under IDEA* (3rd ed.). AOTA Press.

Kielhofner, G. (2008). *Model of human occupation: Theory and application.* Lippincott Williams & Wilkins.

Kiraly-Alvarez, A. (2015). Assessing volition in pediatrics: Using the volitional questionnaire and the pediatric volitional questionnaire. *The Open Journal of Occupational Therapy, 3*(3). https://doi.org/10.15453/2168-6408.1176

Mattingly, C., & Fleming, M. (1994). *Clinical reasoning: Forms of inquiry in therapeutic practice.* F. A. Davis.

Pierce, D. (2001). Untangling occupation and activity. *American Journal of Occupational Therapy, 55,*138-146.

Puchalski, C., Ferrell, B., Virani, R., Otis-Green, S., Baird, P., Bull, J., Chochinov, H., Handzo, G., Nelson-Becker, H., Prince-Paul, M., Pugliese, K., & Sulmasy, D. (2009). Improving the quality of spiritual care as a dimension of palliative care: The report of the Consensus Conference. *Journal of Palliative Medicine, 12*(10), 885-904. https://doi.org/10.1089/jpm.2009.0142

Reid, D., Chiu, T., Sinclair, G., Wehrmann, S., & Naseer, Z. (2006). Outcomes of an occupational therapy school-based consultation service for students with fine motor difficulties. *Canadian Journal of Occupational Therapy, 73,* 215-224.

Rodger, S., & Ziviani, J. (Eds.). (2006). *Occupational therapy with children: Understanding children's occupations and enabling participation.* Blackwell Publishing Ltd

Rogers, J. (1983). Eleanor Clarke Slagle Lecture: Clinical reasoning: The ethics, science and art. *American Journal of Occupational Therapy, 37*(9), 601-616.

Smits-Engelsman, B. C., Blank, R., van der Kaay, A. C., Mosterd-van der Meijs, R., Vlugt-van den Brand, E., Polatajko, H. J., & Wilson, P. H. (2013). Efficacy of interventions to improve motor performance in children with developmental coordination disorder: A combined systematic review and meta-analysis. *Developmental Medicine and Child Neurology, 55*(3), 229-237. https://doi.org/10.1111/dmcn.12008

Swinth, Y., Spencer, K. C., & Jackson, L. L. (2007). Occupational therapy: Effective school-based practices within a policy context. (COPSSE Document Number OP-3). University of Florida, Center on Personnel Studies in Special Education.

Trombly, C. (1993). Anticipating the future: assessment of occupational function. *American Journal of Occupational Therapy, 47*(3), 253-257. https://doi.org/10.5014/ajot.47.3.253

Wehrmann, S., Chiu, T., Reid, D., & Sinclaii, G. (2006). Evaluation of occupational therapy school-based consultation service for students with fine motor difficulties. *Canadian Journal of Occupational Therapy, 73*, 225-235.

Yerxa, E. (1990). An introduction to occupational science: A foundation for occupational therapy in the 21st century. *Occupational Therapy in Health Care, 6*, 1-7.

5

Theory-Based Intervention

Patricia Laverdure, OTD, OTR/L, BCP, FAOTA
and Francine M. Seruya, PhD, OTR/L, FAOTA

Chapter Objectives

1. Describe the ways in which occupational therapy theoretical foundations align with intervention processes outlined in the fourth edition of the *Occupational Therapy Practice Framework: Domain and Process (OTPF-4)*.
2. Examine the influencing factors on practice and the ways they support our role delegation and improve the value of our contributions in school practice.
3. Discover ways to align occupation-based practice with state and core educational standards and high-leverage practices (HLPs).

Theoretical foundations enable us to address explicitly the student's strengths and needs and link them to current and future participation and achievement. Therefore, our theory enables us to leverage strengths, prioritize needs, and establish action steps to effect change. As discussed in the previous chapter, evaluation via the occupational profile; structured, formalized, and standardized assessment; and clinical judgment help the practitioner to identify strengths and challenges as well as begin to select an organizing model of practice by which to understand the student as an occupational being within the school context. Via the initial evaluation, other areas of need may become apparent, thereby creating the need for additional or complementary models of practice to further facilitate the ability to meet the desired outcomes.

Laverdure, P., & Seruya, F. M. *Theory in School-Based Occupational Therapy Practice: A Practical Application* (pp. 61-67). DOI: 10.4324/9781003526773-5

In addition to intervention addressing areas of challenge or barriers identified via the evaluation, the school-based therapist must also consider educational regulations and practices because we need to strive to align our practice with educational standards. We have discussed the importance of professional identity, especially in school settings, and the ability to understand, support, and use the common language of the educational setting will further facilitate the development of this identity as well as help other stakeholders on the educational team see the value of partnering with occupational therapists. Furthermore, working to align interventions and goals to meet the educational standards outlined by state or district requirements is an essential component of contextually based delivery within a school setting.

INTEGRATING EDUCATIONAL LEGISLATION AND PRACTICE

Practicing in educational settings not only requires occupational therapy practitioners to effectively use theory in their clinical reasoning and intervention but also to integrate knowledge of state and federal educational legislation and guidance and school district, school, and classroom culture, procedures, and routines (Swinth et al., 2007). In addition, skillful translation of multidisciplinary research produced largely from either clinical or educational perspectives is necessary (Grajo et al., 2020). Finally, we must balance these influences with the needs of the student, family, instructional staff, school, and school district, rendering unique recommendations to meet the constantly changing demands of the occupations and task demands and the contexts of the school setting.

OCCUPATION-BASED PRACTICE IN ALIGNMENT WITH STATE AND CORE STANDARDS

As discussed in Chapter 3, the American Occupational Therapy Association (AOTA), in its summative document describing the inter-related constructs that describe occupational therapy practice (i.e., the fourth edition of the *OTPF-4*; AOTA, 2020), includes nine areas of occupation of central interest to occupational therapy practitioners: activities of daily living, instrumental activities of daily living, health management, rest and sleep, education, work, play, leisure, and social participation (AOTA, 2020). Engaging in occupations of relevance and meaning provides important opportunities for the development of motor, social, cognitive, and vocational skills for students and can promote positive healthy engagement in social and learning communities (Parham & Fazio, 2008). Additionally, productive participation in meaningful occupations contributes to a student's development of identity, perceptions of competence, sense of health, and well-being (AOTA, 2020). Building skills that enable students to manage their personal needs is essential for autonomy, and these skills are often important prognostic indicators for future employment of individuals (Klinger & Dudley, 2021). When occupational therapy practitioners use an occupation-based theoretical approach, they improve student access to the environment and instruction; establish strategies to leverage strengths and overcome barriers; and improve outcomes for independent living, postsecondary education, and vocational success.

Although these areas of occupation are valuable and directly impact students' ability to effectively participate and make progress in their educational programs, therapists often have difficulty understanding how they align with curricular standards adopted nationally (Common Core State Standards) or by individual state educational agencies (State Standards). Although national and state curricular standards, available through the U.S. Department of Education or state (for those states that have not adopted the Common Core State Standards) departments of education, explicitly outline educational expectations in the areas of reading, math, and writing, they also offer valuable learning expectations across an array of functional skills in these academic as well as life skill areas. However, it can prove difficult for occupational therapy practitioners to articulate areas of priority and align these areas with specific developmental stages, ages, or grade levels at which the progression of skills is expected. Unlike teachers on the team, occupational therapy practitioners often lack clearly identified and standardized developmental/learning progressions as they are identified in core curricular standards and, as a result, may have difficulty describing baseline, identifying specific goals, monitoring progress, and articulating outcomes in a way that clearly aligns with educational standards.

These skill pathways, described in the educational literature as *learning progressions*, provide an organized and sequenced road map that students traverse as they develop and master the skills needed for postsecondary success (Howe et al., 2020). Often aligned with learning standards and grade-level expectations, learning progressions provide team members with valuable information about where the student is on the continuum toward mastery and what skills continue to need support. To align components of the *OTPF-4* and our scope of practice with the learning progressions outlined by educational standards, occupational therapists frequently use theoretical models that are developmentally based to guide their professional reasoning.

Howe and colleagues (2020) posited that occupational therapists may ground their theoretical foundations in occupation-based and developmental theories as a guide to determine a child's current ability in participating in various activities or skills. They discussed developmental models as being stage specific, based on ecological theory, or acquisitionally based. These theories help therapists to critically explore children's development from a multitude of perspectives and integrate the biological, contextual, and behavioral components that lead to skill development. They also provide foundational assumptions that help inform our understanding of the development of skills that support occupational engagement and performance such as the progression of fine motor development, social-emotional learning, and how behavior can be shaped based on experiences with the environment (Howe et al., 2020). School-based occupational therapists frequently use these developmental theories to determine the current level of skill in these domains, and many of the component, skill-based assessments typical in pediatric practice are also based on developmental theories. These developmental progressions can be likened to the learning progressions used in educational settings as part of core curricular outcomes. Although not always aligned explicitly with the standards of learning, these developmental progressions can be a valuable method to evaluate and design intervention when used in conjunction with other theories to focus the child as an occupational being within the school context. Therapists can use their knowledge of development to align specific goal areas with those of the Common Core or other educational guidelines being used within their own school settings.

INTERVENTION ALIGNMENT WITH THE OCCUPATIONAL THERAPY PRACTICE FRAMEWORK: DOMAIN AND PROCESS

The *OTPF-4* identifies diverse types of intervention approaches (AOTA, 2020). Occupational therapy intervention approaches are the "specific strategies selected to direct the evaluation and intervention processes on the basis of the client's desired outcomes, evaluation data, and research evidence" (AOTA, 2020, p. 61). The *OTPF-4* explicitly notes that intervention approaches specifically relate to theoretical practice models and frames of reference (AOTA, 2020). The way in which therapists implement intervention is defined by intervention types, which include "occupations and activities, interventions to support occupations, education and training, advocacy, group interventions, and virtual interventions" (AOTA, 2020, p. 59). Certain approaches and interventions align well with various theoretical bases and will further help the therapist think critically and reason to select appropriate organizing and complementary models (Ikiugu & Smallfield, 2011).

To demonstrate the applicability of theory to various intervention approaches, we present each approach and an example of a theoretical assumption that can be implemented in alignment with the approach. The first intervention approach, creates or promotes, assumes no current disability or builds on the strengths and capacities of the student in each context. The use of reinforcement via a star chart for all children in a kindergarten class to follow the typical classroom schedule would be an example of how the theoretical constructs of a behavioral model or positive mental health could support this type of intervention approach. Establish or restore is an intervention approach that seeks to develop a skill that has either not been developed or was lost because of impairment. Providing range of motion exercises or facilitating typical movement patterns are examples of how the biomechanical or neurodevelopmental treatment frames of reference can be applied to this approach. Maintain is an approach that supports the current developmental status and prevents loss of skill. Working in an ongoing manner to preserve active head range of motion to access an augmentative and alternative communication device would be an example of this approach within the education setting. Modify is an intervention approach that seeks to make changes either to context or task components to allow a student to achieve satisfactory occupational performance. Providing various assistive technology devices such as pencil grips and slant boards could be considered part of the modification approach and draws from the biomechanical theoretical perspective because they seek to support anatomical alignment and the ability to function in both static and dynamic movement patterns. Finally, prevent is an approach that seeks to deter barriers to occupational performance. Using habituation as a part of the Model of Human Occupation to develop routines for a child to complete the morning unpack routine would be an example of the application of theory to this approach.

Likewise, when selecting how a therapist will implement their intervention, the theoretical components of specific models and frames of reference are applicable. Participation is paramount in supporting students in educational settings. Engaging with educational staff to design instruction and interventions to ensure students are active members of the classroom; participating in classroom activities and routines; and successfully fulfilling roles as student, peer, friend, and helper are essential to meeting the goals of public education. Implementing participation-based intervention via occupations and activities aligns well with many of the occupation-based models such as occupational adaptation, the Model of Human Occupation, and the Person-Environment-Occupation model. Each of these models uses occupation-based interventions to address areas of challenge. For example, occupational adaptation posits that an individual can only engage in the process of occupational adaptation to satisfactorily engage in the desired occupation through the act of participating in that desired occupation. Interventions to support occupations include activities used to prepare an individual for participation in occupation. An example of using sensory-based theoretical assumptions is decreasing sensory over-responsiveness via looking for letters in a box of rice to prepare a child for participation in a gluing activity the teacher is implementing to facilitate letter formation.

Further examples of implementing various intervention approaches and types are provided in Chapters 6 through 11 and are more specifically aligned with various occupation-based models and frames of reference as they are applied through the application of organizing and complementary models of practice.

HIGH-LEVERAGE PRACTICES

Drawing from scientific literature across disciplines can support the advancement of effective practice in educational settings. In 2014, an effort was undertaken by the Board of Directors of the Council for Exceptional Children (CEC) to develop a set of highly effective practices aimed at improving the instruction of students with disabilities (Leko et al., 2015; McDonald et al., 2013; McLeskey et al., 2017). The CEC partnered with the Collaboration for Effective Educator Development, Accountability, and Reform (CEEDAR) Center at the University of Florida to establish a team of practitioners, scholars, researchers, teacher preparation faculty, and advocates who developed a list of 22 evidence-based instructional strategies that support student learning and improve outcomes (CEC and CEEDAR Center, 2019a). The strategies, called *HLPs*, are organized into four main overlapping and iterative categories: collaboration; assessment; social/emotional/behavioral practices; and instruction (all areas of critical occupational therapy contribution and all in alignment with the approaches outlined in the *OTPF-4*). McLeskey and colleagues (2017) suggested that although these practices may be helpful for all students, they consist of specially designed intervention strategies to be implemented in unique instructional contexts. Often, the authors suggested, the content of the practices may be substantially different, although it may undergird the achievement of grade-level content or promote successful postsecondary outcomes.

Instructional practices that are based in evidence, applicable across content areas, occur frequently, and can be taught effectively in teacher preparation programs are included in the list of HLPs (McLeskey et al., 2017). The CEC and CEEDAR team members considered practices that focus on effective instruction, prioritize student engagement, and support comprehensive student learning goals. The following are the practices adopted by the CEC and promulgated through their extensive library of resources (CEC and CEEDAR Center, 2019b):

- Collaboration: Teams collaborate to ensure that educational programs effectively meet the needs of students with disabilities.
  - Collaborate with professionals to increase student success.
  - Organize and facilitate effective meetings with professionals and families.
  - Collaborate with families to support student learning and secure needed services.
- Assessment: School team members identify the strengths and needs of their students and demonstrate knowledge and skill in assessment methods and analysis of data for effective decision making.
  - Use multiple sources of information to develop a comprehensive understanding of a student's strengths and needs.
  - Interpret and communicate assessment information with stakeholders to collaboratively design and implement educational programs.
  - Use student assessment data, analyze instructional practices, and make necessary adjustments that improve student outcomes.

- Social/emotional/behavioral: Team members work to create learning environments that are consistent, organized, and promote student success and well-being.
  - Establish a consistent, organized, and respectful learning environment.
  - Provide positive and constructive feedback to guide students' learning and behavior.
  - Teach social behaviors.
  - Conduct functional behavioral assessments to develop individual student behavior support plans.
- Instruction: Team members are knowledgeable about the general education curriculum, curricular standards, learning progressions, and evidence-based practices and skilled in applying this knowledge to prioritize student learning goals and designing and delivering instruction.
  - Identify and prioritize long- and short-term learning goals.
  - Systematically design instruction toward specific learning goals.
  - Adapt curriculum tasks and materials for specific learning goals.
  - Teach cognitive and metacognitive strategies to support learning and independence.
  - Provide scaffolded supports.
  - Use explicit instruction.
  - Use flexible grouping.
  - Use strategies to promote active student engagement.
  - Use assistive and instructional technologies.
  - Provide intensive instruction.
  - Teach students to maintain and generalize new learning across time and settings.
  - Provide positive and constructive feedback to guide students' learning and behavior.

With a focus on occupation and guided by occupation-based theoretical foundations, occupational therapy practitioners can make substantive contributions to students, the team, schools, and school districts in support of the four HLPs. Likewise, the HLPs offer us an evidence-based pathway to support effective instructional strategies and approaches that, when used collaboratively and deliberately, can help students achieve the skills necessary for a successful future. The HLPs offer us a pathway to share our expertise; collaborate to effect change; and facilitate powerful approaches to evaluation, intervention planning and intervention, and instruction delivery that can boost our influence for students, the classroom, and the entire school community.

CONCLUSION

Adopting occupation-based theoretical foundations in school practice guides evaluation, decision making, and intervention planning and empowers occupational therapy practitioners with the tools to identify students' strengths and needs and link them to current and future participation and achievement. As discussed in this chapter, our theoretical foundations and subsequent occupation-focused practice enabled us to leverage strengths, prioritize needs, and establish action steps to effect change in the ever-changing landscape of public schools. Considering occupation and the occupational interests and needs of our students within the context of the school setting and in alignment with core educational standards enables us to respond effectively and integrate educational legislation, sociopolitical perceptions of health and wellness, occupational therapy theory and evidence, and educational best practices into our theory-based intervention planning and implementation. As discussed in the following chapters, using occupation-based theoretical foundations to guide our practice enables us to consider our students' occupational engagement across each of the domains of occupation (AOTA, 2020) and supports the engagement of our full scope of practice.

Using data collected through our evaluation as described in Chapter 4, we can develop interventions that are distinctly tailored to the student's individual strengths, needs, values, and interests and prioritize actions that are not only valuable for the student but also are necessary for the student's active participation in school, home, and community environments. Guided by our theoretical foundations, we integrate the varying perspectives of the student, teacher, and family members and determine how strengths of the student, their educational team, and the environments in which they engage can be leveraged to mediate the barriers to participation. Placing our theoretical foundations at the center of this process equips us with the opportunity to serve not only as decision makers for and with our clients but also as occupational "choice offerers" (Mattingly & Fleming, 1994) by placing value on the students' role as advocates and architects of their future; the family members' role as providers of care, values, and culture; the educators' role as teachers of meaningful experience; and our role as imagineers of possibilities (vs. generators of probabilities). In Chapters 6 through 11, we more explicitly examine the process of how to apply an organizing model of practice to develop a student's occupational profile, discuss strengths and needs, and explore complementary models of practice to uncover additional supports and resources needed to support team decision making and develop an intervention plan for the student (Ikiugu & Smallfield, 2011).

REFERENCES

American Occupational Therapy Association. (2020). Occupational therapy practice framework: Domain and process (4th ed.). *American Journal of Occupational Therapy, 74*(Suppl. 2), 7412410010p1-7412410010p87. https://doi.org/10.5014/ajot.2020.74S2001

Council for Exceptional Children and Collaboration for Effective Educator Development, Accountability, and Reform Center. (2019a). *Analyzing high-leverage practices: Current status*. https://highleveragepractices.org/sites/default/files/2020-10/Analyzing-High-Leverage-Practices-Current-Status-2.pdf

Council for Exceptional Children and Collaboration for Effective Educator Development, Accountability, and Reform Center. (2019b). *High-leverage practices in special education: Overview*. https://highleveragepractices.org/sites/default/files/2020-10/Overview.pdf

Grajo, L. C., Laverdure, P., Weaver, L. L., & Kingsley, K. (2020). Becoming critical consumers of evidence in occupational therapy for children and youth. *The American Journal of Occupational Therapy, 74*(2), 7402170020p1-7402170020p7. https://doi.org/10.5014/ajot.2020.742001

Howe, T. S., Kramer, P., & Hinojosa, J. (2020). Developmental perspective: Fundamentals of developmental theory. In P. Kramer, J. Hinojosa, & T. S. Howe (Eds.), *Frames of reference for pediatric occupational therapy* (4th ed., pp. 20-27). Wolters Kluwer.

Ikiugu, M., & Smallfield, S. (2011). Ikiugu's eclectic method of combining theoretical conceptual practice models in occupational therapy. *Australian Occupational Therapy Journal, 58*(6), 437-446. https://doi.org/10.1111/j.1440-1630.2011.00968.x

Klinger, L. G., & Dudley, K. M. (2021). Interventions to support transition to adulthood for individuals with autism spectrum disorder. In F. R. Volkmar (Eds.), *Encyclopedia of autism spectrum disorders*. Springer. https://doi.org/10.1007/978-3-319-91280-6_102314

Leko, M., Brownell, M., Sindelar, P., & Kiely, M. (2015). Envisioning the future of special education personnel preparation in a standards-based era. *Exceptional Children, 82*, 25-43.

Mattingly, C., & Fleming, M. H. (1994). *Clinical reasoning: Forms of inquiry in a therapeutic practice*. F. A. Davis.

McDonald, M., Kazemi, E., & Kavanaugh, S. (2013). Core practices of teacher education: A call for a common language and collective activity. *Journal of Teacher Education, 64*, 378-386.

McLeskey, J., Barringer, M.-D., Billingsley, B., Brownell, M., Jackson, D., Kennedy, M., Lewis, T., Maheady, L., Rodriguez, J., Scheeler, M. C., Winn, J., & Ziegler, D. (2017, January). *High-leverage practices in special education*. Council for Exceptional Children & CEEDAR Center. https://highleveragepractices.org/wp-content/uploads/2017/06/Preface.Intro1_.pdf

Parham, D., & Fazio, L. (2008). *Play in occupational therapy for children* (2nd ed.). Elsevier, Inc.

Swinth, Y., Spencer, K. C., & Jackson, L. L. (2007). Occupational therapy: Effective school-based practices within a policy context (COPSSE Document Number OP-3). University of Florida, Center on Personnel Studies in Special Education.

6

Activities of Daily Living and Instrumental Activities of Daily Living

Patricia Laverdure, OTD, OTR/L, BCP, FAOTA
and Deborah Schwind, DHSc, OTR/L, BCP, SCSS, FAOTA

Chapter Objectives

1. Define the occupations of activities of daily living (ADLs) and instrumental activities of daily living (IADLs) and describe the ways in which these occupations are experienced in school by students.
2. Identify the ways in which the occupations of ADLs and IADLs align with the purpose and requirements of public school education.
3. Describe the ways in which occupational therapy practitioners evaluate and establish intervention plans grounded in theory for students with needs in the areas of ADLs and IADLs.

ADLs and IADLs are essential occupations that form the foundation for engagement in meaningful roles and routines across the life span (American Occupational Therapy Association [AOTA], 2020; Beisbier & Laverdure, 2020; Laverdure & Beisbier, 2021). ADLs are the personal care activities that we perform on a daily basis to manage the care and nurturance of our bodies (e.g., eating, feeding, toileting, bathing and grooming, dressing), and IADLs are those activities that support the everyday care needs that occur in the home or in the community (e.g., care of others and pets, home management, meal preparation, safety management, financial management; AOTA, 2020).

In school settings, the development of ADL and IADL skills is closely aligned to the Individuals with Disabilities Education Act (IDEA, 2004)–identified priorities for independent living, postsecondary education, and employment. Although academics are of central concern in school settings,

Laverdure, P., & Seruya, F. M. *Theory in School-Based Occupational Therapy Practice: A Practical Application* (pp. 69-85). DOI: 10.4324/9781003526773-6

IDEA recognizes that ADL and IADL skill development promotes independence and provides a foundation for meaningful civic and employment engagement after high school. Functional and independent living skills can be hallmarks for later success (Mazzotti et al., 2021). Students who are independent with ADL and IADL skills have improved educational, independent living, and productive employment outcomes (Pillay & Brownlow, 2017; Rowe et al., 2015; Test et al., 2009).

ADLs and IADLs are characterized by cultural differences that inform expectations, assignments, and motivation for participation (Coppens et al., 2016) and represent a key developmental activity and important predictor of postsecondary success for children and youth (Mazzotti et al., 2016). Youth who regularly perform ADLs and IADLs report higher levels of self-efficacy, task orientation, competence, and self-direction across contexts (Riggio et al., 2010). When there is less independence with ADLs and IADLs, there is decreased quality of life and increased health care usage (Spillman, 2004). Therefore, addressing skills in these areas is imperative and aligns with the scope of occupational therapy practice in schools. Research indicates the following:

- Children are more willing to perform ADLs and IADLs if motivating routines and consistent expectations are established (Klein & Goodwin, 2013; Rende, 2014).
- Engagement in ADLs and IADLs promotes the skills required for self-regulation, task mastery, responsibility, and accountability (Riggio et al., 2010), foundational executive function prerequisites.
- Executive functioning improves academic achievement and successful school outcomes (Ahmed et al., 2018; Willoughby et al., 2019). If a student has the executive functioning skills to complete multistep tasks, they may be able to learn other relevant independent and employment tasks (Ohio Employment First, 2020).
  - Many of the IADL tasks also correlate specifically with employment opportunities. For example, if a student can feed a pet, they may be able to work for a veterinarian, on a farm, in a pet store, or for a dog walking business. If a student can make their own bed or do laundry, they may be able to work in a spa, resort, hospital, or long-term care facility. If they can make coffee, they may be able to work as a barista. If they can make a sandwich, they may be able to work in a restaurant.
- Successful performance of ADLs and IADLs can impact self-esteem and quality of life (Haber et al., 2016), skills essential for postsecondary education success.
  - If a student can set their alarm, eat healthy, manage their health and medications, manage their dorm room and personal interactions (including conflicts), and navigate the campus, they may be more successful in college.
- It is critical that ADL and IADL skill development begin as early as possible to build the foundational skills young adults will need to be successful in their postsecondary environments (Laverdure et al., 2021; Schwind et al., 2021) and can be addressed by occupational therapy practitioners as part of their domain and practice (Carroll & Schwind, 2023).
  - Students with physical disabilities may have difficulties with these occupations, and it is imperative that strategies (e.g., systematic instruction for motor planning and coaching), adaptations (e.g., visuals for sequencing steps), and modifications (e.g., engagement in varying activities) be provided.
  - Students with cognitive and memory impacts or attention and impulsivity may need systematic instruction and scaffolds (e.g., cognitive supports, visual cues, video modeling, cognitive applications [apps]) in ADLs and IADLs for independent performance (Baer et al., 2011; Cobb et al., 2013; Rabren et al., 2002).

IDEA requires that postsecondary transition planning begin by age 16 years, although there are many states that recognize that transition be addressed by age 14 years to effect positive student outcomes. Those states that address transition by age 14 years have better employment outcomes because the students have more time to develop ADLs, IADLs, and employment skills (Haber et al., 2016). One of the best predictors of success upon graduation is whether a student has volunteer work, internships, or paid work while in high school (Mazzotti et al., 2021; Shogren, 2011; Wehman et al., 2014). If independent living, which includes ADL and IADL tasks, can predict successful outcomes, it is essential that occupational therapy practitioners address these skills while students are in school to ensure success upon graduation.

ACTIVITIES OF DAILY LIVING AND INSTRUMENTAL ACTIVITIES OF DAILY LIVING IN THE SCHOOL SETTING

The occupations associated with ADL and IADL routines are a part of a student's everyday life in school settings. Students unpack their backpacks, take off and hang their coats, and organize their school materials. They use the restroom, manage toileting hygiene tasks (e.g., clean the perineal area), and perform other hygiene-related tasks (e.g., wash hands, comb hair). They manage clothing and clothing closures after use of the restroom, before and after recess, when readying for physical education, and when organizing for dismissal. At lunch or snack, students open a variety of containers, carry their lunch tray, swipe their card and/or enter their identification number, and manage utensils. Throughout the day, they manage many mobility opportunities across environments on various surfaces (e.g., getting on or off the bus, walking around obstacles in the classroom, walking in line, running on the playground and in physical education, climbing stairs) and maintain static positions (e.g., standing upright, sitting in a desk chair, sitting on stools, sitting on the floor) requiring coordination, motor planning, endurance, and strength. They also engage in numerous positional changes (e.g., move from floor to stand, stand to sit in chair, stand to sit on bench in cafeteria).

Occupational therapy practitioners are instrumental in supporting the development of ADL and IADL skills in school and use a variety of evidence-based interventions that fall within our scope of practice (Alwell & Cobb, 2009; Beisbier & Laverdure, 2020; Cobb & Alwell, 2009; Laverdure & Beisbier, 2021; Laverdure et al., 2021). There is strong evidence that using an occupation-based intervention approach and promoting ADL and IADL participation in authentic contexts effectively promotes ADL and IADL performance. Occupational therapy practitioners can begin to address foundational ADL and IADL skills in preschool. Structured pretend and imaginary play and dress-up activities can develop important ADL and IADL skills and promote role exploration and perspective taking. Preschoolers can play in helper stations, making toast as a parent, scooping ice cream in the ice cream shop, or placing plates in the restaurant as a waiter. They can take on the role of doctor, nurse, or veterinarian and address health maintenance occupations. Spaces can be designed to promote the roles of car mechanic or hairstylist. In their play with life roles, they are learning, sequencing, and practicing the steps of ADLs and IADLs and adapting and modifying their performance through problem solving, decision making, and self-determination. Their success with these activities is reinforced socially through their social interactions with peers and their increasing mastery. Pretend play engagement is limited for children with disabilities (Amaral et al., 2014; Guichard & Grande, 2018; Lavesser & Berg, 2011; Law et al., 2013), and developing opportunities for students to successfully engage is essential.

In elementary school, there are numerous ADL performance expectations that include donning, doffing, and hanging one's coat; managing personal belongings (e.g., backpack, lunch bag, books, materials); and unpacking and packing for the day's activities. Lunch routines require competencies in carrying a tray, using utensils, opening containers, feeding oneself, and cleaning up one's space. Students participate in classroom (e.g., maintain an organized classroom, manage classroom tools and resources, manage the classroom pet) and school-based (e.g., newscaster on the news show, safety patrol, flag raiser, library helper, preschool helper, technology helper, table wiper, sweeper, agenda collector, mail collector, pencil sharpener, chair stacker) jobs that promote the development of ADL and IADL skills. Although the amount of assistance required to complete ADLs and IADLs is proportional to the complexity of the health care needs, developmental impairment, and neurobehavioral symptomatology (Amaral et al., 2014; Dunn & Gardner, 2013; Dunn et al., 2009), through participation in these activities, children with disabilities develop skills essential for self-efficacy and adult success at home, in the community, and in future work environments (Gall et al., 2006).

As they move to middle and high school, ADL and IADL responsibilities expand. Students change for physical education. They may shower, especially if they are on an athletic team or club. Occupational therapy practitioners must consider and implement the modifications and adaptations required to promote successful engagement in these valuable occupations. Are they able to use their visual perceptual skills to don their clothes correctly? Do they need adapted shoelaces so they can put their shoes on in a timely manner? Can they navigate the lock on the locker in the locker room? In middle and high school, they may be taking Career and Technical Education classes including Family and Consumer Science (FACS), Technical Education, Computer Technology, Art, Music, Band, and Drama. These classes expose them to not only increasingly complex ADL and IADL responsibilities but also new role, routine, and career options. For example, in FACS, students may learn to cook, shop, devise a healthy meal, sew, and manage laundry. Classes such as FACS are important and provide hands-on opportunities for students to explore different life skills and careers to better align interests and strengths with employment training and participation. By experiencing some of these activities in a hands-on way, students may be able to self-express personal goals for self-determination and self-advocacy (Schwind et al., 2021).

Throughout their school years, students may have the opportunity to participate in a community-based instruction (CBI) program. CBI is an evidence-based strategy that promotes the generalization of skills from the classroom to a real-life setting, and research shows that it increases success upon graduation (Wehman et al., 2014). CBI often incorporates functional reading, math, and writing; safety; and money skills. CBI is generally performed off campus and includes activities such as navigating public transportation or visiting a grocery store or restaurant. However, CBI can also be performed in the school where the school serves as the community, and it can begin earlier in a student's educational program, providing repetition and practice needed for success. In this way, the size of the community and the complexity of the activity are modified for success.

Numerous school-based CBI activities have been developed and may include taking care of a class or school pet; managing a school garden, compost, or bird feeder; operating a school lost and found; or operating a school ice cream stand. When all students participate in the school-based CBI program, a sense of community and belonging, self-esteem, and self-determination are facilitated, along with the development of essential IADL skills for the future (Schwind et al., 2021). School-based CBI programs are inclusive and promote problem solving through the application of skills in a real-life context. Performing IADLs alongside their general education peers can develop empathy and understanding (Schwind et al., 2021).

CBI may also include school-based enterprises that can begin in elementary school and expand through middle and high school. Examples include the following:

- The farmer's market: Students can work in the school garden and sell their harvested crops at a school-sponsored farmer's market. The farmer's market can expand in middle and high school to include more items, more days, a larger garden, a larger stand, and higher dollar amounts. They can create and sell flower arrangements.

- The school store: Middle and high school students can operate a school store or coffee shop. They can make and sell dog bones or flavored popcorn, have a florist shop, and so on.

These activities require and promote IADL skills and provide the opportunity to generalize literacy, math, communication, and social skills; improve workplace behaviors; and develop self-determination. With careful grading, practice, and reinforcement, these early school-based CBI experiences may lay the foundation for generalizing IADL skills to an off-campus location that supports the transition to competitive employment. Framing CBI as a continuum and progression in this way allows us to increase duration and steps, expand responsibilities, and increase independence.

As occupational therapy practitioners, we can provide strategies and suggestions, adaptations, and modifications while students are engaged in work simulation and internships as well. There are many opportunities to build and reinforce ADL and IADL skill development and performance. Analyzing, adapting, and modifying occupations, materials, and environments to ensure success are key contributions we make to the student and their team. Employing an occupational analysis approach, we identify the following (AOTA, 2020; Thomas, 2023):

- What occupations are relevant to the student? What ADL and IADL skills can promote the most valuable long-term outcomes? In what occupations is the student most interested?
- What are the materials and tools that the student will need to access and use? Can they lift it, carry it, and manipulate it? What adaptations are necessary for effective use?
- What are the requirements of the physical space and social environment for effective occupational engagement? What training and resources will be required to ensure success?
- What performance skills are required for successful participation? Can the student coordinate and move themselves and the objects in the environment effectively to engage in the occupation? Can the student effectively attend to the task? Can they follow directions and organize and sequence steps? Can they manage their time, and can they complete the task without error? Can they solve problems that they might encounter, and can they ask for help when needed?
- What client factors are required for safe and successful participation? What sensory, motor, cognitive, communicative, and motivational factors are required?

Recognizing the critical value of ADL and IADL skills to productive living after high school empowers our responsibility to participate in curriculum development, adapt materials, and modify occupation to promote student access, participation, and success. By (a) incorporating explicit and systematic instruction from the earliest opportunity, (b) providing evidence-based interventions and scaffold (e.g., coaching and hierarchical prompting, visual and video supports, simulation, social stories), (c) building opportunity for practice and repetition in natural contexts, (d) expanding complexity and requirements for generalization, and (e) collaborating with school team members and caregivers, we set students up for positive outcomes after school (Alwell & Cobb, 2009; Beisbier & Laverdure, 2020; Cobb & Alwell, 2009; Laverdure & Beisbier, 2021; Rende, 2014). We must consider the following:

- How are we engaging students in ADLs and IADLs throughout their school day?
- Are we modifying their ADL and IADL responsibilities and adapting the tasks to promote access and enhance participation and performance at the earliest opportunity (e.g., preschool, kindergarten, primary school)?
- Are we helping students explore career options and express their career interests and preferences in multiple ways (e.g., digital book, video)?
  - Do you like performing outdoor or inside chores?
  - Do you like performing chores alone or with other people?
  - Would you rather cook in a quiet kitchen or busy kitchen?

- Are students able to generalize IADL skills learned in school-based CBI to off-campus CBI experiences?
- Are we building connections for careers that may be associated with IADL tasks they enjoy?

CASE STUDY

Jane is an 8-year-old student with Down syndrome who attends her neighborhood elementary school. At the end of her preschool year, her eligibility for special education services was reevaluated, and an occupational therapy evaluation was completed. The occupational therapy evaluation consisted of observation in a variety of school settings to include the preschool classroom, the cafeteria, and the playground. Observation of Jane's transition to and from the school bus and into the classroom as well as opportunities to transition through the school building were observed. Functional skills assessments to address fine and gross motor, ADL, and IADL skills were performed. The Peabody Developmental Motor Scales was administered. The results of the occupational therapy evaluation were aggregated with observations and assessments of other school team members and observation and concerns of her caregivers, and she was found eligible for special education services under the educational disability category of intellectual disability (a change from developmental disability).

Jane is currently placed in a first-grade classroom that is cotaught by the classroom and special education teachers. As the team prepares for her next eligibility reevaluation, the occupational therapist considers Jane's previous occupational therapy evaluation, her progress over the last 3 years, and Jane's occupational profile (AOTA, 2020). Table 6-1 reflects Jane's occupational profile as she nears the end of first grade.

Organizing Model of Practice: Person-Environment-Occupation and Person-Environment-Occupation-Performance Model

Jane's occupational profile highlights a mismatch between her occupational performance and the interests that she must engage in in meaningful ways with occupations of interest and the environment. As a result, the Person-Environment-Occupation (PEO) model (Baum et al., 2015) was chosen as the organizing model of practice (Ikiugu & Smallfield, 2011). The PEO model began to take shape in the late 1980s and early 1990s, at a time in the history of occupational therapy's prolific advancement of its theoretical foundations (particularly those that focused on holistic and client-centered approaches), the expansion of ideas around the use of clinical reasoning in the occupational therapy process (Mattingly & Fleming, 1994; Rogers, 1983), and the emergence of occupational science constructs (Yerxa, 1990). Informed by similar ideas, the Person-Environment-Occupation-Performance (PEOP) model quickly followed, and the two models gave rise to a deeper understanding of occupation as the essential functions that people need and want to do to engage in their daily lives. The expansion of these ideas occurred while occupational therapy practitioners, rich in theoretical practice underpinnings in mechanistic, reductionistic, and biomedical views of occupational therapy practice, entered educational practice in response to the passage of Public Law 94-142, the Education for All Handicapped Children Act. Originally posited as a "transactive approach to occupational performance" (Law et al., 1996, p. 12), PEO and PEOP are grounded in the following:

- Psychosocial and neurobehavioral models that focus on factors in the environment that influence behavior and learning in individuals (Lawton & Nahemow, 1973; Moos, 1980)

TABLE 6-1

Jane's Occupational Profile

What concerns do Jane and her team have about her occupational engagement?	Jane has difficulty managing ADL and IADL tasks at home and school. She has difficulty problem solving during complex tasks. Her endurance is weak, and her motor skills are delayed.
In what occupations is Jane successful, and what barriers impact her success?	Jane enjoys participating in school-based CBI and exclaims that it is her favorite part of the school day. ADL and IADL task components involving memory, problem solving, sequencing, strength, and endurance are difficult. Her verbal communication is not easily understood. She needs frequent rests throughout her day and needs adaptation of fine and gross motor tasks.
What is Jane's occupational history?	Jane is independent in basic ADL using visual supports. She enjoys her role as student in the classroom and art class but is challenged by reading and drawing. She enjoys recess. Jane began participating in school-based CBI this school year and expresses interest in engaging in more school tasks.
What are Jane's and her team's personal interests and values?	Jane enjoys interacting and playing games with her peers. She enjoys having a peer read to her. She actively interacts with her family and friends after school. She engages in Girl Scouts, swims on a swim team with modifications, and participates in an after-school cooking club that incorporates health habits such as yoga. In the summer, she participates in hippotherapy.
	(continued)

TABLE 6-1 (CONTINUED)
Jane's Occupational Profile

What aspects of the contexts do Jane and her team see as supporting engagement in desired occupations, and what aspects are inhibiting engagement?

	SUPPORTING	INHIBITING
ENVIRONMENT	She has a large peer group in the fully inclusive general education classroom with special education support, a large accessible playground, classroom jobs, and a school-based CBI program. She uses an alternative and augmentative communication (AAC) device.	Jane is challenged by poor safety awareness. She has exhibited eloping behaviors from the classroom and the playground.
PERSONAL	Jane is well liked and accepted by her family and peers. She is a hard worker and enjoys engaging in activities she finds meaningful.	Jane's intelligence quotient is 65. She is beginning to be able to identify some letters and requires her academic work to be modified. Her physical, emotional, and cognitive stamina is limited, and she fatigues easily.
PERFORMANCE PATTERNS	Jane has become independent with her arrival, dismissal, and lunch routines using visual schedules outlining task steps. She fulfills roles of daughter, sister, student, friend, and worker (in CBI).	

What client factors do Jane and her team see as supporting engagement in desired occupations, and what aspects are inhibiting engagement?

	SUPPORTING	INHIBITING
VALUES, BELIEFS, AND SPIRITUALITY	Jane has a large, supportive, and loving family that has realistic expectations for her ADLs and IADLs in the future. She is actively engaged in her church and attends religious classes that are modified for her.	She can exhibit challenging behaviors due to frustration as well as decreased physical, emotional, or cognitive stamina.
BODY FUNCTIONS	Jane is involved in activities that promote physical activity and ADL/IADL independence.	She has memory challenges, delayed cognitive processing, and difficulty following multistep directions. She can become easily frustrated with academic activities. Jane has low muscle tone and reduced stamina.
BODY STRUCTURES	When using her AAC device, Jane can pair two words in communication.	Jane has strabismus and wears glasses. She has poor fine, gross, and oral motor coordination. She has poor speech intelligibility. Jane has issues with constipation. She is at risk for weight issues in the future.

(continued)

TABLE 6-1 (CONTINUED)	
Jane's Occupational Profile	
What are Jane's and her team's priorities and desired goals?	
OCCUPATIONAL PERFORMANCE	Jane has a strong desire to interact with her peers and perform a variety of functional ADL and IADL tasks that demonstrate her strengths. She wants to be a contributor to her social and learning environment.
PREVENTION	Jane's team wants to reduce her frustration with challenging tasks, reduce her eloping behaviors, and increase her safety.
HEALTH AND WELLNESS	Jane and her family want her to maintain an active lifestyle (activity and healthy eating) to both mitigate her risk of weight gain as well as decrease challenges with constipation.
QUALITY OF LIFE AND WELL-BEING	Jane, her family, and her school team want to continue her progression toward ADL and IADL independence to increase her outlooks for postsecondary living and employment success.
PARTICIPATION AND ROLE COMPETENCE	Jane enjoys school-based jobs with modifications for her motor control and is interested in having more school and home responsibilities.
OCCUPATIONAL JUSTICE	Jane, her family, and her school team want to ensure that she has the skills to be successful and participate in her community.

Adapted from American Occupational Therapy Association. (2020). AOTA occupational profile template. https://www.aota.org/-/media/Corporate/Files/Practice/Manage/Documentation/AOTA-Occupational-Profile-Template.pdf

- Ecological systems theory models commonly used in child development structures that examine "fit" between the individual and the environment (Bronfenbrenner, 1977, 1989; Kahana, 1982)
- Global health care and public health models that support change efforts in environmental affordances and barriers to enhance wellness and quality of life (Howe & Briggs, 1982; Weisman, 1981; World Health Organization, 2001)

The models examine the complex relationship between person, environment, occupation, and occupational performance factors and how the affordances and barriers within and between these components influence performance, participation, and quality of life (Baum et al., 2015). Central to the work of occupational therapy practitioners in the educational environment is the need to address and mitigate the person, occupation, environment, and occupational performance challenges facing students, their caregivers, and the educational system in which they participate. Baum and colleagues (2015) argued that "Occupational therapy is the bridge between the medical system where the person receives diagnosis-based care and the sociocultural level of care where the person receives interventions relevant to everyday living" (p. 50). In educational settings, occupational therapy practitioners bridge both the medical and educational systems in which the student receives diagnosis-based care (identified as both medical or educational deficits) and the participation-based care in which the student receives interventions that promote access, participation, and belonging. The models became important theoretical tools for occupational therapy practitioners who were searching to articulate the ways in which we maximize occupational performance in occupations of value to students and the environments in which they participate. The PEO and PEOP models not only allow occupational therapy practitioners a means to examine the variety of influential factors on access and participation, but they also allow us to examine how these factors influence development over the life span.

The key domains of the PEO and PEOP models are person, environment, occupation, and occupational performance (in PEOP), and using the models allows us to use the language of the fourth edition of the *Occupational Therapy Practice Framework: Domain and Process* (AOTA, 2020) in articulating our domain and value to the educational team.

The person describes the personal characteristics of the student, and the model postulates that the person is capable of accessing and participating in occupations, routines, and roles that they need and want to do and that performance will change in relation to the occupations and environments with and in which they participate.

The environment refers to the "contexts and situations which occur outside of the individual and elicit responses from them" (Law, 1991, p. 175). Environments and contexts can influence client factors, occupations, and occupational performance. Environmental barriers are one of the first things often considered by occupational therapy practitioners practicing in educational settings.

Occupation is considered both the ordinary, routine, habitual, taken-for-granted parts of our daily lives as well as the special parts of our lives that carry symbolic meaning. It includes the nine areas of occupation identified in the domain of occupational therapy (AOTA, 2020).

Occupational performance is the "doing of meaningful activities, tasks, roles through complex interactions between the person and the environment" (Baum et al., 2015, p. 52). Occupational performance skills (motor, process, and social interaction) and performance patterns (habits, rituals, routines, and roles) as well as occupational priorities shift and change continually across time and space in relation to the growth and development of the student as well as the occupational, contextual, and environmental demands on them.

Using the PEO model as a guiding theoretical framework, the occupational therapist gathered data regarding Jane's strengths and needs. Using structured observation across the contexts that she participates in, the strengths and challenges that impact Jane's ADL and IADL performance and participation were identified (Table 6-2). In addition, a measure that assesses a student's performance of functional activity in school, the School Function Assessment, was administered (Coster et al., 1998). The School Function Assessment is a judgment-based (questionnaire) assessment tool that is used to measure a student's ability to perform functional tasks that support participation in the academic and related social aspects of an educational program for children in kindergarten through sixth grade. Criterion scores range from 0 to 100 and were developed on a population of students with disabilities. Criterion cutoff scores indicate how students perform compared to general education peers. For each task area, a cutoff score for that domain indicates the expected range of performance. The data collected confirmed the theoretical assumptions of the organizing model of practice.

Complementary Models of Practice

The occupational therapist determined that to more fully understand Jane's strengths and challenges related to her motor performance, additional information was required. The acquisitional frame of reference (FOR) and motor control and learning theories were chosen as complementary models of practice.

TABLE 6-2

Jane's Strengths and Challenges

COMPONENT	STRENGTHS	CHALLENGES
Person	• High interest and engagement in ADL and IADL tasks • Motivated to achieve mastery in ADL and IADL tasks	• Easily frustrated by multistep ADL and IADL tasks • Requires structure, cues, and reinforcement for participation • Has decreased stamina for physical and cognitive tasks
Environment	• Well-supported and inclusive environment • Participation in class-based CBI	• Needs close supervision in the environment because of eloping behaviors
Occupation	• Independent in basic ADLs with visual cues and schedule • Opportunity for repetition, practice, and generalization of skills in home, school, and community	• Requires assistance with toileting routines (managing clothing closures, toileting hygiene, and washing hands) • Requires assistance with lunch routines (opening packages and cleaning up) • Requires assistance with tasks that require three or more steps

Acquisitional Frame of Reference

The acquisitional FOR was developed by Dr. Anne Mosey as a reflection of her belief that occupational therapy is "an action oriented experience [in which] clients learn by doing" (Lewis, 2003, p. 9). In alignment with Jane's strong interest in interacting in her environment, the acquisitional FOR purports that learning occurs when individuals interact with a reinforcing environment through repetition and practice (Luebben & Royeen, 2010). This complementary model of practice was chosen because of its focus on the mastery of skills required for optimal participation in life roles and routines and its particular focus on motor and cognitive skills. In addition, although the acquisitional FOR promotes skill development through practice, it does not suggest that skill acquisition is necessarily sequential, which aligns with cognitive and motor developmental profiles observed in children with Down syndrome (Kim et al., 2017). Instead, it suggests that skills stand alone and that the environment is a significant determinant of behavior and skill development (Luebben & Royeen, 2010). The acquisitional FOR emphasizes functional skills and learned behaviors, and the quality of the performance is not the main focus, particularly in the beginning of skills development. Self-care skills are often a primary area of skill development addressed in the acquisitional FOR, and, as in the case of Jane, the mastery of these skills can be intrinsically motivating, promoting improved performance and generalization (Luebben & Royeen, 2010).

In the acquisitional FOR, activity and occupational analyses are central to the promotion of learning and development. Thomas (2023) describes activity analysis as the identification of the demands of an activity as it is typically done and occupational analysis as the ways that the individual engages in that activity in a way that represents their own roles, routines, and context. Activity and occupational analyses are used to determine what skills need to be performed (identification of goals); the client factors; environmental factors, body functions, and performance required for successful engagement in the occupation; how to break down the specific steps and sequences (teaching strategy); and the promotion of generalization to other contexts such as the use of different objects while engaging with different individuals and engaging in different settings (Luebben & Royeen, 2010).

Jane was highly motivated to engage in activities and occupations that her peers were engaged in. She was motivated by participation in ADLs and IADLs, and using the acquisitional FOR, we were able to identify and prioritize tasks of interest, conduct thorough task analyses, and teach skills that she would engage in and practice. Through this process, Jane mastered and generalized valuable skills required for successful participation in school, home, and community environments.

Motor Control and Learning Theories

In addition, motor control and learning theories consider the neuromaturational aspects of motor development and consider the predictable sequences of motor development and skilled volitional movement. Although a number of motor control and learning theories exist, they represent the evolution of biomechanical and neuromaturational theories and FORs that explain how the motor system is controlled (Cole & Tufano, 2019). Motor control and learning theories apply principles of physics and physiology as well as neurology to human movement. They illustrate the ways in which skilled volitional movement is influenced by reflex hierarchical or neuromaturational sequence controlled by the central nervous system, that movement control occurs in a cephalocaudal and proximal to distal orientation, and that movement involves both feedback and feed-forward loop mechanisms (Cole & Tufano, 2019). In addition, engaging clients in meaningful activity provides motivation for increased effort and practice, attributes for the development and refinement of proximal and postural control, and attributes for the development of gross and fine motor skill.

In Jane's case, motor control theory was chosen to address her proximal motor control; strengthen her postural control for endurance; promote mobility and gross motor control; and improve her reach, grasp, and manipulation skills. The occupational therapist administered the Goal-Oriented Assessment of Lifeskills (Miller et al., 2013) to assess Jane's functional motor skills required for ADL and IADL performance. Understanding the influence of Jane's motor system capacities and deficits enabled the occupational therapist to prioritize her needs and develop her goals, intervention approaches, and plan. Because of Jane's interest in and motivation for participation in ADL and IADL tasks, using motor control and learning theories to adapt the environment and identify meaningful and functional motor skill challenges and client-centered goals was appropriate and relevant for her educational program participation.

Because of Jane's reduced muscle tone and endurance and the delay in the development of motor skills and control, efforts to develop environmental modifications to provide adequate proximal support both in sitting and for manipulating school tools and resources were developed (e.g., a supportive chair for her desk, seating for circle time, adapted toilet seat for toileting, adapted tools for writing and art, an adapted tool for self-care [e.g., zipper pulls]). Activities that promote proper positioning, strength, and endurance were incorporated throughout her school day. For example, Jane was highly motivated to write on the board, so many of her writing activities were completed on an easel in the classroom.

We chose an instructive and strategy-based motor control and learning theory approach that focused on her recognition of her goals, tasks, and regulatory cues through demonstration. We strengthened her knowledge of her performance through feedback during performance and with regard to goal achievement (Leech et al., 2021). We established opportunities for task repetition using the school and home environments and the objects within them; created learning progressions as described in Chapter 4; and provided verbal, visual, and manual feedback. We gradually created opportunities for Jane to practice new skills in a variety of environments, promoting carryover and generalization to novel environments.

Goals and Interventions

Using a top-down approach, ADLs and IADLs are identified as both intervention and expected outcomes. The occupational therapist collaborated with Jane's team to prioritize areas of highest need and formulated goals addressing the development of ADL and IADL skills (Table 6-3). Furthermore, using engagement in ADLs and IADLs of Jane's interest and choosing, the occupational therapist collaborated with the team to identify the specific engagement opportunities and instructional strategies (e.g., explicit routines and role-playing, visual schedules/cues, social stories, interactive books, video modeling, school-based CBI) that would be used to support Jane's engagement and practice. In addition, the occupational therapist collaborated with Jane's family to build awareness of the value and hierarchical development of home chores. Occupational performance, role competence, and participation were identified as Jane's occupational therapy outcomes.

Although these may be tasks that could be addressed by an educational team including an occupational therapy practitioner, there would not be this many goals related to ADL or IADL tasks. This serves to provide ideas for the multitude of goals that an occupational therapy practitioner could support in the educational environment related to ADL and IADL tasks.

TABLE 6-3

Jane's Activities of Daily Living and Instrumental Activities of Daily Living Goals and Intervention Plan

OCCUPATION	GOAL (PERSON)	ENVIRONMENTAL/ACTIVITY ADAPTATION/MODIFICATION
Toileting	Will be independent with the toileting routine to include handwashing	Visual schedule Visual cues
Hygiene	Will be independent with the handwashing routine	Visuals, depress paper towel dispenser
Dressing	Will be independent with a variety of clothing closures	Buttons on coat, hang up coat, tie shoes, use button bags at centers, work in lost and found (CBI)
Feeding	Will be independent during lunch with packaging	Opening packages
Functional mobility	Will perform a task requiring physical activity for more than 10 minutes independently	Using cart in building or standing to perform a school-based job (CBI) Motor planning sitting at cafeteria table, sitting on floor, and getting up
Care of others/ community	Will complete a three-step classroom or school-based task independently	Compost, food recovery, water plants, feed birds (CBI)
Care of pets	Will work with peer to complete a classroom or school-based task	Feed turtles or the birds (CBI)
Communication management	Will self-advocate when she needs help using the AAC device or to charge the AAC device	Charge AAC, care of AAC, use on news show, ask for help
Community mobility	Will navigate the building independently to participate in school-wide CBI program	Library job (CBI)
Financial management	Will sort more than five different items independently	School store to sort items (CBI) Sort coins and bills (CBI)
Health management	Will choose a self-regulation strategy from a playlist or menu and will then complete a task independently	Pushing, lifting, body parts for hurt, self-regulation
Home establishment and management	Will complete three classroom or school-based jobs	Vacuum, sweep, wipe tables (CBI)
Meal preparation and cleanup	Will sort more than five different items independently	Food recovery (CBI), after-school cooking club
Safety/emergency maintenance	Will self-advocate when she needs help using the AAC device	Fire drill, tornado drill, ask for help
Shopping	Will sort more than five different items independently	Lemonade stand, farmer's market, school store (CBI)

Adapted from American Occupational Therapy Association. (2020). Occupational therapy practice framework: Domain and process (4th ed.). *American Journal of Occupational Therapy, 74*(Suppl. 2), 7412410010p1-7412410010p87. https://doi.org/10.5014/ajot.2020.74S2001

CONCLUSION

Meeting the needs of students in the occupational areas of ADLs and IADLs is paramount because participation, performance patterns, and performance skills in these areas form an important foundation for engagement in meaningful roles and routines across the life span. In addition, skill performance and perception of competence are closely aligned with long-term educational priorities for independent living, postsecondary education, and employment. As noted, participation in these fundamental occupations is cornerstone to the achievement of developmental motor, social, emotional, and academic growth; engagement in functional activities in the home, school, and community; participation in school-related tasks and school routines; and readiness for postsecondary goal accomplishment. Occupational therapy practitioners bring their unique lens to the challenges students experience in ADLs and IADLs and create effective interventions that not only improve performance but also create opportunities for students to build their skills for their future. In the next chapter, we build on these concepts and introduce the occupation of health management. We examine occupation-based theoretical foundations that support the design and implementation of occupation-based evaluation and intervention approaches for health management in school settings.

REFERENCES

Ahmed, S. F., Tang, S., Waters, N. E., & Davis-Kean, P. (2018). Executive function and academic achievement: Longitudinal relations from early childhood to adolescence. *Journal of Educational Psychology, 11*, 446-458. https://doi.org/10.31234/osf.io/xd5jy

Alwell, M., & Cobb, B. (2009). Functional life skills curricular interventions for youth with disabilities. *Career Development for Exceptional Individuals, 32*(2), 82-93.

Amaral, M. F. D., Drummond, A. F., Coster, W. J., & Mancini, M. C. (2014). Household task participation of children and adolescents with cerebral palsy, Down syndrome and typical development. *Research in Developmental Disabilities, 35*(2), 414-422. https://doi.org/10.1016/j.ridd.2013.11.021

American Occupational Therapy Association. (2020). Occupational therapy practice framework: Domain and process (4th ed.). *American Journal of Occupational Therapy, 74*(Suppl. 2), 7412410010p1-7412410010p87. https://doi.org/10.5014/ajot.2020.74S2001

Baer, R. M., Daviso, A. W., Flexer, R. W., Queen, R. M., & Meindl, R. S. (2011). Students with intellectual disabilities: Predictors of transition outcomes. *Career Development for Exceptional Children, 34*, 132-141.

Baum, C., Christiansen, C., & Bass, J. (2015). The Person-Environment-Occupation-Performance model. In C. Baum, C. Christiansen, & J. Bass (Eds.), *Occupational therapy: Performance, participation, and well-being* (4th ed., pp. 49-56). SLACK Incorporated.

Beisbier, S., & Laverdure, P. (2020). Occupation and activity-based interventions to improve performance of instrumental activities of daily living and rest/sleep for children and youth aged 5-21: A systematic review. *American Journal of Occupational Therapy, 74*(2), 7402170042.

Bronfenbrenner, U. (1977). Toward an experimental ecology of human development. *American Psychologist, 32*, 513-530.

Bronfenbrenner, U. (1989). Ecological systems theory. *Annals of Child Development, 6*, 187-249.

Carroll, T. C., & Schwind, D. (2023). Practice improvement per: Evidence-based predictors of post-school success. *OT Practice, 28*(8).

Cobb, R., & Alwell, M. (2009). Transition planning/coordinating interventions for youth with disabilities. *Career Development for Exceptional Individuals, 32*(2), 70-81.

Cobb, R. B., Lipscomb, S., Wolgemuth, J., Schulte, T., Veliquette, A., Alwell, M., Batchelder, K., Bernard, R., Hernandez, P., Holmquist-Johnson, H., Orsi, R., Sample McMeeking, L., Wang, J., & Weinberg, A. (2013). *Improving post-high school outcomes for transition-age students with disabilities: An evidence review (NCEE 2013-4011).* National Center for Education Evaluation and Regional Assistance, Institute of Education Sciences. http://ies.ed.gov/ncee/pubs/20134011/pdf/20134012.pdf

Cole, M., & Tufano, R. (2019). *Applied theories in occupational therapy* (2nd ed.). SLACK Incorporated.

Coppens, A., Alcala, L., Rogoff, B., & Mejia-Arauz, R. (2016). Children's contribution in family work: Two cultural paradigms. In S. Punch & R. M. Vanderbeck (Eds.), *Families, intergenerationality, and peer group relations, geographies of children and young people* (pp. 1-28). Springer. https://doi.org/10.1007/978-981-4585-92-7_11-2

Coster, W., Deeney, T., Haltiwanger, J., & Haley, H. (1998). *School functional assessment.* Pearson Education, Inc.

Dunn, L., Coster, W. J., Orsmond, G. I., & Cohn, E. S. (2009). Household task participation of children with and without attentional problems. *Physical & Occupational Therapy in Pediatrics, 29*(3), 258-273. https://doi.org10.1080/01942630903008350

Dunn, L., & Gardner, J. (2013). Household task participation of children with and without physical disability. *American Journal of Occupational Therapy, 67*(5), e100-e105. https://doi.org/10.5014/ajot.2013.00812

Gall, C., Kingsnorth, S., & Healy, H. (2006). Growing up ready: A shared management approach. *Physical & Occupational Therapy in Pediatrics, 26*(4), 47-62. https://doi.org/10.1080/J006v26n04_04

Guichard, S., & Grande, C. (2018). Differences between pre-school children with and without special educational needs functioning, participation, and environmental barriers at home and in community settings: An international classification of functioning, disability, and health for children and youth approach. *Frontiers in Education, 3*, 7. https://doi.org/10.3389/feduc.2018.00007

Haber, M., Mazzotti, V., Mustian, A., Rowe, D., Bartholomew, A., Test, D., & Fowler, C. (2016). What works, when, for whom, and with whom: A meta-analytic review of predictors of postsecondary success for students with disabilities. *Review of Educational Research, 86*(1), 123-162.

Howe, M., & Briggs, A. (1982). Ecological systems model for occupational therapy. *American Journal of Occupational Therapy, 36*, 322-327.

Ikiugu, M., & Smallfield, S. (2011). Ikiugu's eclectic method of combining theoretical conceptual practice models in occupational therapy. *Australian Occupational Therapy Journal, 58*(6), 437-446. https://doi.org/10.1111/j.1440-1630.2011.00968.x

Individuals with Disabilities Education Act of 2004, Pub. L. No. 108-446, § 118 Stat. 2647 (2004).

Kahana, E. (1982). A congruence model of person-environment interaction. In M. P. Lawton, P. G. Windley, & T. D. Beyers (Eds.), *Aging and the environment: Theoretical approaches* (pp. 97-121). Springer.

Kim, H. I., Kim, S. W., Kim, J., Jeon, H. R., & Jung, D. W. (2017). Motor and cognitive developmental profiles in children with Down syndrome. *Annals of Rehabilitation Medicine, 41*(1), 97-103. https://doi.org/10.5535/arm.2017.41.1.97

Klein, W., & Goodwin, M. H. (2013). Chores. In E. Ochs & T. Kremer-Sadlik (Eds.), *Fast-forward family: Home, work, and relationships in middle-class America* (pp. 130-148). University of California Press.

Laverdure, P., & Beisbier, S. (2021). Occupation- and activity-based interventions to improve performance of activities of daily living, play, and leisure for children and youth ages 5 to 21: A systematic review. *American Journal of Occupational Therapy, 75*, 7501205050. https://doi.org/10.5014/ajot.2021.039560

Laverdure, P., Nemec, E., Johnson, C., & Blake, T. (2021). Evaluating interventions that improve participation in chores in children and youth with disabilities: A systematic review. *Journal of Occupational Therapy, Schools, & Early Intervention, 14*(3), 257-273. https://doi.org/10.1080/19411243.2021.1875384

Lavesser, P., & Berg, C. (2011). Participation patterns in preschool children with an autism spectrum disorder. *Occupation, Participation and Health, 31*(1), 33-39. https://doi.org/10.3928/15394492-20100823-01

Law, M. (1991). The environment: A focus for occupational therapy. *Canadian Journal of Occupational Therapy, 58*, 171-179.

Law, M., Anaby, D., Teplicky, R., Khetani, M. A., Coster, W., & Bedell, G. (2013). Participation in the home environment among children and youth with and without disabilities. *British Journal of Occupational Therapy, 76*(2), 58-66. https://doi.org/10.4276/030802213X13603244419112

Law, M., Cooper, B., Strong, S., Stewart, D., Rigby, P., & Letts, L. (1996). The Person-Environment-Occupation Model: A transactive approach to occupational performance. *Canadian Journal of Occupational Therapy, 63*(1), 9-23.

Lawton, M., & Nahemow, L. (1973). Toward an ecological theory of adaptation and aging. In W. Preiser (Ed.), *Environmental design research* (pp. 24-32). Dowden, Hutchison & Ross.

Leech, K. A., Roemmich, R. T., Gordon, J., Reisman, D. S., & Cherry-Allen, K. M. (2021). Updates in motor learning: Implications for physical therapist practice and education. *Physical Therapy, 102*(1), pzab250. https://doi.org/10.1093/ptj/pzab250

Lewis, S. C. (2003). *Elder care in occupational therapy* (2nd ed., p. 9). SLACK Incorporated.

Luebben, A. J., & Royeen, C. B. (2010). An acquisitional frame of reference. In P. Kramer & J. Hinojosa (Eds.), *Frames of reference for pediatric occupational therapy* (3rd ed., pp. 461-488). Lippincott Williams & Wilkins.

Mattingly, C., & Fleming, M. (1994). *Clinical reasoning: Forms of inquiry in therapeutic practice.* F. A. Davis.

Mazzotti, V., Rowe, D., Kwiatek, S., Voggt, A., Chang, W., Fowler, C., Poppen, M., Sinclair, J., & Test, D. (2021). Secondary transition predictors of postschool success: An update to the research base. *Career Development and Transition for Exceptional Individuals, 44*(1), 47-64.

Mazzotti, V. L., Rowe, D. A., Sinclair, J., Poppen, M., Woods, W. E., & Shearer, M. L. (2016). Predictors of post-school success. *Career Development and Transition for Exceptional Individuals, 39*(4), 196-215. https://doi. org/10.1177/2165143415588047

Miller, L. J., Oakland, T., & Herzberg, D. S. (2013). Goal-Oriented Assessment of Life Skills (GOAL). WPS.

Moos, R. (1980). Specialized living environments for older people: A conceptual framework for evaluation. *Journal of Social Issues, 36,* 75-94.

Ohio Employment First. (2020). *Evidence based predictors for post-school success: Ohio Employment First transition framework evidence based predictors tool.* https://ohioemploymentfirst.org/up_doc/Evidence_Based_ Predictors_for_Post_school_Success3_25_15.pdf

Pillay, Y., & Brownlow, C. (2017). Predictors of successful employment outcomes for adolescents with autism spectrum disorders: A systematic literature review. *Review Journal of Autism and Developmental Disorders, 4,* 1-11. https://doi.org/10.1007/s40489-016-0092-y

Rabren K., Dunn C., & Chambers D. (2002). Predictors of post-high school employment among young adults with disabilities. *Career Development for Exceptional Individuals, 25,* 25-40.

Rende, R. (2014). The developmental significance of chores: Then and now. *The Brown University Child and Adolescent Behavior Letter, 31*(1), 1-7. https://doi.org/10.1002/cbl.30009

Riggio, H. R., Valenzuela, A. M., & Weiser, D. A. (2010). Household responsibilities in the family of origin: Relations with self-efficacy in young adulthood. *Personality and Individual Differences, 48*(5), 568-573. https://doi.org/10.1016/j.paid.2009.12.008

Rogers, J. (1983). Eleanor Clarke Slagle Lecture: Clinical reasoning: The ethics, science and art. *American Journal of Occupational Therapy, 9,* 601-616.

Rowe, D. A., Alverson, C. Y., Unruh, D. K., Fowler, C. H., Kellums, R., & Test, D. W. (2015). A Delphi study to operationalize evidence-based predictors in secondary transition. *Career Development and Transition for Exceptional Individuals, 38,* 113-126. https://doi.org/10.1177/2165143414526429

Schwind, D., Orlin, M., Davidson, L., & Kaimal, G. (2021). Evaluating a novel approach to community based instruction. *Journal of Occupational Therapy, Schools and Early Intervention.* https://doi.org/10.1080/19411 243.2021.1910609

Shogren, K. (2011). Culture and self-determination: A synthesis of the literature and directions for future research and practice. *Career Development for Exceptional Individuals, 34*(2), 115-127.

Spillman, B. C. (2004). Changes in elderly disability rates and the implications for health care utilization and cost. *Milbank Quarterly, 82,* 157-194. https://doi.org/10.1111/j.0887-378X.2004.00305.x

Test, D., Fowler, C., Richter, S., White, J., Mazzotti, V., Walker, A. R., Kohler, P., & Kortering, L. (2009). Evidence-based practices in secondary transition. *Career Development for Exceptional Individuals, 32*(2), 115-128.

Thomas, H. (2023). *Occupation-based activity analysis* (3rd ed.). SLACK Incorporated.

Wehman, P., Schall, C., Carr, S., Targett, P., West, M., & Cifu, G. (2014). Transition from school to adulthood for youth with autism spectrum disorder. *Journal of Disability Policy Studies, 25*(1), 30-40.

Weisman, G. D. (1981). Modeling environment-behavior systems: A brief note. *Journal of Man-Environment Relations, 1,* 32-41.

Willoughby, M. T., Wylie, A. C., & Little, M. H. (2019). Testing longitudinal associations between executive function and academic achievement. *Developmental Psychology, 55,* 767-779. https://doi.org/10.1037/ dev0000664

World Health Organization. (2001). *International Classification of Functioning, Disability and Health.* Author.

Yerxa, E. (1990). An introduction to occupational science: A foundation for occupational therapy in the 21st century. *Occupational Therapy in Health Care, 6,* 1-7.

7

Health Management

Patricia Laverdure, OTD, OTR/L, BCP, FAOTA
and Tammy Blake, OTD, OTR/L

Chapter Objectives

1. Define the occupation of health management and describe the ways in which this occupation is experienced in school by students.
2. Identify the ways in which the occupation of health management aligns with the purpose and requirements of public school education.
3. Describe the development of health management curricula and the ways in which occupational therapists address health management in school settings.
4. Describe the ways in which occupational therapy practitioners use theory to evaluate and establish intervention plans for students with needs in the area of health management.

The fourth edition of the *Occupational Therapy Practice Framework: Domain and Process*, an official document of the American Occupational Therapy Association (AOTA), describes health management as an occupation focused on "developing, managing, and maintaining health and wellness routines, including self-management, with the goal of improving or maintaining how to support participation and other occupations" (2020, p. 32). The occupation of health management includes (a) the management of conditions and symptoms, medication, nutritional needs, and personal care devices; (b) physical, social, and emotional health promotion; and (c) the communication of health care needs with the health care team (AOTA, 2020). Health management and occupational

Laverdure, P., & Seruya, F. M. *Theory in School-Based*
Occupational Therapy Practice: A Practical Application (pp. 87-100).
DOI: 10.4324/9781003526773-7

participation are integrally related and result collectively in the improvement of one's quality of life. Attending to one's health care needs maximizes the capacity to participate in occupations that are desired and meaningful and promote health and wellness.

ROLE OF OCCUPATIONAL THERAPY IN HEALTH MANAGEMENT

Using a variety of intervention types, occupational therapy practitioners help clients to adapt and modify their involvement in occupations to promote healthy lifestyle choices; prevent and/or minimize illness, injury, or disability; and/or facilitate adaptation and recovery from disease or injury (AOTA, 2015). In a school setting, occupational therapy practitioners support numerous hygiene and safety initiatives commonly undertaken in public schools and collaborate with instructional staff to modify and deliver instruction on health management promotion. For example, the Centers for Disease Control and Prevention (CDC) and the National Education Association provide guidance on advancing hygienic practices in schools that include handwashing, coughing, and sneezing (CDC, 2022a; National Education Association, 2021). Numerous self-care and hygiene programs are commercially available that address topics such as personal appearance, hygiene, body growth and development, and personal safety (Bastian et al., 2014; Wrobel, 2003). In addition, local, state, and federal educational and justice agencies and private foundations have addressed school safety by promoting school climate and positive mental health, threat assessment and mitigation, physical and cybersecurity resources, bullying and violence, and emergency planning (Heritage Foundation, 2022; National Institute of Justice, 2018; SchoolSafety, 2022; U.S. Department of Education Office of Elementary and Secondary Education, 2022).

NATIONAL HEALTH EDUCATION STANDARDS

In 1995, the CDC established the National Health Education Standards (NHES) to establish criteria for health education that increased health-promoting behaviors among students in U.S. public schools (CDC, 2019). Written by a coalition of professionals represented by the American Public Health Association, the American School Health Association, the American Association for Health Education, and the CDC, the coalition argues that the characteristics of an effective health education curriculum include instructing students in essential and functional knowledge of health and health management and developing individual and group personal values, beliefs, norms, and skills to adopt, practice, and maintain healthy behaviors and lifestyle (CDC, 2019). The NHES has adopted standards that address the following:

* Comprehension of concepts related to health promotion and disease prevention
* Influence of family, peers, culture, media, technology, and other factors on health behaviors
* Ability to access valid information, products, and services to enhance health
* Use of interpersonal communication skills to enhance health and avoid or reduce health risks
* Use of decision-making and goal-setting skills to enhance health
* Ability to practice health-enhancing behaviors and avoid or reduce health risks
* Ability to advocate for personal, family, and community health

To advance alignment between the public health and education sectors, the CDC in collaboration with Association for Supervision and Curriculum Development, a private educational nonprofit organization, launched the Whole School, Whole Community, Whole Child (WSCC) model in 2014 to improve students' cognitive, physical, social, and emotional development through school health initiatives (CDC, 2022b). The WSCC model encompasses physical activity and education, nutrition services, health education, social and emotional climate, physical and mental health services, family engagement, community involvement, and employee health. The CDC and Association for Supervision and Curriculum Development brought together leaders from an array of fields to include health, public health, education, and school health to design a collaborative approach to improve health learning across the nation. Many states have used the NHES standards and the WSCC model to develop health curricula that include topics such as understanding body systems, physical and mental health, social and emotional wellness, nutrition, disease prevention and health promotion, safety and injury prevention, substance abuse prevention, and community and environmental health.

In school settings, occupational therapy practitioners leverage their expertise in health and wellness to advance students' knowledge and skills in health management throughout their elementary, middle, and high school years. Table 7-1 illustrates the trajectory of health management concepts that are supported by occupational therapy.

CASE STUDY

Arnez is a 10-year-old only child who lives with his mother and father and paternal grandmother. He had an unremarkable perinatal, prenatal, and medical history and began to sit alone at 12 months old, walk at 18 months old, and babble at 24 months old. He has been exposed to both Kurdish and English languages, and his parents indicate he understands both languages. At 2.5 years of age, he underwent a speech and language evaluation at an outpatient pediatric clinic because of his parent's concerns for his expressive and receptive language and hearing. His parents reported he did not talk much at home, and his primary means of communication was gesturing. The results of the evaluation revealed a moderate to severe expressive and receptive language disorder and mild hearing loss.

After the evaluation, he was referred to his school district for an evaluation and was later found eligible for special education services because of developmental delays across all domains of development. An Individualized Education Program (IEP) was developed that focused on Arnez's receptive and expressive language, preacademic, and motor skill development. He began receiving special education services through half-day class-based preschool and Head Start. After sharing the school evaluation with his pediatrician, Arnez was seen for further diagnostic testing and was diagnosed with mitochondrial encephalopathy, a rare genetic disorder that affects all organs of the body, particularly the central nervous system and muscles, of children beginning between the ages of 2 and 10 years. Mitochondrial encephalopathy is a progressive disorder that can cause muscle weakness and impaired coordination, fatigue, hearing and vision loss, heart and kidney problems, severe headaches and seizures, anorexia and vomiting, diabetes, and hormonal imbalances. There is no known cure for mitochondrial encephalopathy; treatment is experimental and palliative and consists of enzymes, amino acids, antioxidants, and vitamins. The disease results in early mortality.

TABLE 7-1

Health Management Concepts Across the Grade Levels

GRADE LEVEL	CONCEPTS
Kindergarten	• Recognize basic facts about the body • Manage basic hygiene responsibilities such as toileting and handwashing • Regulate social and emotional responses • Follow school safety rules • Seek assistance from trusted adults
1	• Understand the body's major organs • Understand the impact of behavior on health and wellness (consequences) • Develop respect for self and others (self and social awareness) • Explore concepts of responsible decision making
2	• Understand the body's structures and functions • Develop knowledge of illness and disease prevention (nutrition and substance use) • Engage in responsible decision making
3	• Understand the impact of healthy habits on growth and development • Application of the knowledge of health risk reduction and healthy behavioral choices • Understand the impact of personal health decisions on oneself and others
4	• Understand concepts of disease prevention • Develop skills and resilience to substance abuse • Assume responsibility for decision making relative to health
5	• Distinguish reliable from unreliable health information and resources • Assume responsibility for healthy habits and decision making • Engage in behaviors that promote healthy lifestyles
6	• Apply knowledge of physical, emotional, social, and environmental health to personal and family health behavior habits • Understand adolescent health issues • Engage in injury prevention behaviors
7	• Understand the relationship between healthy lifestyle, effective interpretation of health information, and good health outcomes • Choose positive alternatives to risky behaviors • Resist peer pressure • Manage stress and anxiety
8	• Understand the origins and causes of diseases • Interpret and apply consumer information to promote healthy behaviors and lifestyle • Engage in health behaviors that address specific personal, family, and community health concerns

(continued)

TABLE 7-1 (CONTINUED)	
Health Management Concepts Across the Grade Levels	
GRADE LEVEL	**CONCEPTS**
9	• Apply knowledge of health concepts to plan for personal, lifelong health goals • Engage actively in establishing a healthy lifestyle for themselves and advocating for health within their families and communities
10	• Demonstrate comprehensive health and wellness knowledge and skills • Engage in behaviors that maintain good personal health through the life span

Adapted from Health Education Standards of Learning for Virginia Public Schools. (2020). https://doe.virginia.gov/testing/sol/standards_docs/health/index.shtml

During his preschool years, Arnez made slow progress, and as he transitioned to kindergarten, he was reevaluated to determine his ongoing need for special education services. He was again found eligible for services under the educational category of "other health impairment" with delays noted in the areas of cognitive, communication, social/emotional, motor, and adaptive skills development. The goals on his IEP focused on participation in classroom tasks, expressive communication and speech sound production, number and letter recognition, and prewriting skills. The IEP team noted Arnez's increasing difficulty with manipulation of small objects, imitating prewriting strokes, and drawing pictures and determined that additional information was needed to effectively plan for his services. He was subsequently referred for an occupational therapy evaluation. His occupational therapy evaluation revealed weaknesses in fine motor and visual motor skill development, effective hand and tool use, following directions, and completing tasks. Occupational therapy services were added to address these and previously mentioned weaknesses, to support his access to and participation in school routines and activities, and to promote his health management.

Currently, Arnez is in the fourth grade. His medical condition is considered stabilized on medications that are focused on reducing lactic acidosis, epilepsy, cardiac arrhythmia, and malnutrition and normalizing muscle tone. He wears glasses and hearing aids. He has continued to show progressive loss of motor control and uses a power wheelchair to navigate the classroom. He requires periodic breaks for rest because of his fatigue. He has made some progress in reading and math, and he is accessing his education with the supports and scaffolds within his IEP. He continues to require extensive support in math and reading, written expression, expressive communication skills, and movement. Table 7-2 reflects Arnez's occupational profile as a fourth grade student.

TABLE 7-2

Arnez's Occupational Profile

What concerns do Arnez and his team have about his occupational engagement?	Arnez requires assistance to manage all activities of daily living (ADLs), instrumental activities of daily living (IADLs), and health management tasks at home and school. He fatigues easily and gives up when tasks become difficult. As his disease progresses, his parents and school team members note that he requires additional support to access the school building and classroom. He needs increasing support to participate in school and home activities. The team expresses concern for his transition to middle school.
In what occupations is Arnez successful, and what barriers impact his success?	Arnez enjoys watching his peers in the classroom and on the playground. He enjoys playing the symbol in music class and participates in the after-school band program 1 day per week.
What is Arnez's occupational history?	Arnez requires assistance with all school routines and tasks. He is no longer able to negotiate around obstacles in the classroom or longer distances in the hallways or the playground in his power chair. He needs longer rests away from the classroom.
What are Arnez's and his team's personal interests and values?	Arnez enjoys being with his peers in the classroom and enjoys having the teacher or a peer read to him. He interacts with his peers in music/band. He is no longer able to go to Boy Scouts because of his fatigue after school, but his peers often FaceTime (Apple) with him during the Boy Scout meetings.

(continued)

TABLE 7-2 (CONTINUED)

Arnez's Occupational Profile

What aspects of the contexts do Arnez and his team see as supporting engagement in desired occupations, and what aspects are inhibiting engagement?

	SUPPORTING	INHIBITING
ENVIRONMENT	Arnez has a large peer group in the fully inclusive general education classroom with special education support. He accesses the cafeteria and the music room. He uses a power wheelchair, although he needs additional support through tight obstacles and longer distances.	Arnez's fatigue and complex health needs restrict his access to the home, school, and community environments.
PERSONAL	Arnez is well liked and accepted by his family and peers. As his disease has progressed, his family has grown increasingly concerned for his health management and participation.	Arnez's fatigue and medical condition limit his participation. Limited endurance, cognitive involvement, and time away from the classroom are impacting his progress.
PERFORMANCE PATTERNS	Arnez requires assistance with arrival, dismissal, and lunch routines. He needs periodic rest periods away from the class. He needs scaffolds and support for all school tasks and routines. He struggles to maintain being an active participant in the roles of son, student, and friend.	

What client factors do Arnez and his team see as supporting engagement in desired occupations, and what aspects are inhibiting engagement?

	SUPPORTING	INHIBITING
VALUES, BELIEFS, AND SPIRITUALITY	Arnez has a supportive and loving family that has realistic expectations for his health management in the future.	Because of his declining health status and reduced participation, Arnez is increasingly detached from his family and peers.
BODY FUNCTIONS	Frequent breaks support his fatigue and enhance his participation.	He has delayed cognitive processing and difficulty following multistep directions. He is easily fatigued and requires schoolwork to be broken into small tasks.
BODY STRUCTURES	Arnez uses glasses, hearing aids, and a power wheelchair to support his declining body functions. He has a highly active medical team that has used a cocktail of medications to treat his condition, resulting in stabilization of some of his symptoms.	Arnez's progressive disease has resulted in challenges with lactic acidosis, epilepsy, cardiac arrhythmia, malnutrition, and muscle tone.

(continued)

TABLE 7-2 (CONTINUED)
Arnez's Occupational Profile

What are Arnez's and his team's priorities and desired goals?	
OCCUPATIONAL PERFORMANCE	Arnez has a strong desire to interact with his peers and perform a variety of functional school roles, routines, and tasks.
PREVENTION	Arnez's team wants to reduce the demands on his neuromuscular system and provide adequate breaks that maximize his participation in school tasks.
HEALTH AND WELLNESS	Arnez and his family want to maintain his stable condition on the cocktail of medications, resting accommodations, and scaffolds and resources that support his participation in school.
QUALITY OF LIFE AND WELL-BEING	Arnez's family members are aware of his progressive condition and are realistic about the rates of mortality of his condition. They want to ensure his comfort and maximize his participation in school.
PARTICIPATION AND ROLE COMPETENCE	Arnez wants to be an active participant in school, music/band, and Boy Scouts.
OCCUPATIONAL JUSTICE	Arnez, his family, and his school team want to ensure that he can participate maximally in roles, routines, tasks, and activities.

Adapted from American Occupational Therapy Association. (2020). AOTA occupational profile template. https://www.aota.org/-/media/Corporate/Files/Practice/Manage/Documentation/AOTA-Occupational-Profile-Template.pdf

Organizing Model of Practice: Synthesis of Child, Occupational Performance, and Environment In Time Model

Our analysis revealed that Arnez's current and future occupational participation was significantly impacted by his progressive neuromuscular condition. Although motivated to succeed, Arnez fatigues very easily and needs frequent breaks throughout his day. He learns at a slower pace and requires additional time to process and recall information and a wait time before beginning a task and answering questions and participating in and completing tasks. Increasing challenges with occupational performance (e.g., age and grade expectations, motor and cognitive deficits), motivation and psychological needs (e.g., autonomy, relatedness, occupational competence), and current and future contexts (e.g., classroom and school building obstacles, longer distances, changing middle school classrooms) influenced all areas of occupation. To address the complexity of this student's need, we chose an occupation-based organizing model of practice (Ikiugu et al., 2009) that enabled us to consider the influence of Arnez's health condition on his psychological needs, development, and occupational engagement.

The Synthesis of Child, Occupational Performance, and Environmental In Time (SCOPE-IT) model addresses the influence of the student's personal and environmental factors on ever-evolving and developing childhood occupations (Haertl, 2010; Poulsen, 2011; Poulsen & Ziviani, 2004). The SCOPE-IT relies on occupation as both means and ends to improve occupational performance and participation and is based on the following key assumptions (Haertl, 2010; Poulsen, 2011):

- Occupation is the underlying foundation of occupational therapy.
- Children are occupational and social beings, and participation in occupational therapy promotes change and influences health and well-being.
- Occupational performance is influenced by personal, environmental, social, cultural, and temporal factors, and development is influenced by guided participation and innate drive.

Like the Person-Environment-Occupation model discussed in Chapter 6, the fit between the child, environment, and occupation is central; however, in the SCOPE-IT model, the developmental sequence of skill development and student autonomy, competence, and relatedness is considered and leveraged to increase participation and performance (Poulsen et al., 2006). Interventions maximize child-environment-occupation fit by educating and collaborating with the client, caregivers, and instructors to (a) address occupational performance issues, (b) adapt occupations through task analysis and assistive technology, and (c) modify the environment (Poulsen & Ziviani, 2004). Balancing these interventions improves occupational performance, participation, physical and emotional health, and well-being (Ziviani & Poulsen, 2017).

Using the SCOPE-IT model as a guiding theoretical framework, the occupational therapist gathered data regarding Arnez's strengths and needs. Using structured observation across the contexts that she participates in, the strengths and challenges that impact his ADLs, IADLs, education, work/productivity, leisure, rest/sleep performance, and participation were identified. In addition, the Goal-Oriented Assessment of Lifeskills, a measure that assesses a student's performance of functional activity in school, was administered (Miller et al., 2013). The Goal-Oriented Assessment of Lifeskills is an individually administered evaluation of fundamental motor abilities needed for daily living in students 7 to 17 years old. Standard scores have a mean of 100 and a standard deviation of 15. In addition, the School Setting Interview (SSI) was administered (Hemmingsson et al., 2005). The SSI uses a client-centered interview to assist the occupational therapist in intervention planning. The SSI considers the student's occupational performance in all environments in which they assume the student role, including the classroom, playground, gymnasium, corridors, and field trips. The SSI is a semistructured interview designed to assess student-environment fit and identify the need for accommodations for students with disabilities in the school setting. The data collected confirmed the theoretical assumptions of the organizing model of practice and are described in Table 7-3.

Complementary Models of Practice

Given the complexity of Arnez's progressive medical condition, two additional complementary models of practice were selected to address his health management needs, provide additional assessment data, and guide intervention planning (Ikiugu et al., 2009). The first complementary model of practice was the rehabilitative frame of reference (FOR), and the second was the compensatory FOR (Gillen, 2014).

Rehabilitative Frame of Reference

The rehabilitative FOR deepens the understanding of the medical condition, psychological needs, and occupational performance and participation for children with medically complex conditions who are not likely responsive to remediation and guides evaluation and therapeutic intervention.

TABLE 7-3

Arnez's Strengths and Challenges

COMPONENT	STRENGTHS	CHALLENGES
Original participation	• Developmental readiness for autonomy in ADLs, IADLs, education, work/productivity, leisure, and rest/sleep occupations • Follows a familiar set of directions/routines • Progressive neuromuscular disorder stabilized	• Does not perform to age-level expectations • Requires assistance with all occupations • Requires maximal assistance for health management • Works slowly and requires many repetitions/practice • Easily fatigued during occupational performance
Psychological needs (motivation, autonomy, relatedness, and competence)	• Motivated to attempt and participate in all activities • Motivated to achieve mastery in occupations	• Lack of autonomy in occupational participation • Increasing disconnection and relation with peers and classroom (role as student and friend) • Limited feelings of personal competence
Environment	• Uses powered mobility to access his home, school, and community spaces	• Increasing complex environment with greater number of obstacles • Increasing distances to traverse in the school and community • Increasing needs for assistive technology

---

The rehabilitative FOR guides environmental and occupational adaptation, compensation, and environmental modification and promotes occupational participation despite ongoing impairments (Gillen, 2014). The key theoretical assumption underlying the rehabilitative FOR is that clients can achieve satisfying occupational engagement despite persistent challenges in occupational performance. Using the rehabilitation FOR, evaluation and intervention focus on (a) the strengths and capabilities of the client and maximizing the full potential of those strengths and (b) designing compensatory and adaptive measures to enhance function in areas of occupational interest.

The rehabilitation FOR was chosen as the first complementary model of practice for several reasons. First, few people on the education team possessed the practice knowledge of Arnez's complex medical condition to translate its relevance to learning access and participation and to support the management of his health while at school. We used our knowledge of the condition to discuss Arnez's functional skills, to identify expected functional trajectories and goals, and to establish effective instructional and intervention plans to address his complex needs. The rehabilitation FOR guided our collaboration with Arnez's medical team. We also used the rehabilitation FOR to identify, in collaboration with Arnez and his team, Arnez's strengths to determine ways we could enhance his strengths to support his participation in school and home occupations. One such strength that we used was Arnez's strong social relationships with his peers. We established peer partnerships to support Arnez's access to the environment and the materials within it. His peers took turns collecting his needed materials and bringing them to him. We found this strategy was able to preserve Arnez's endurance and increase his time in the classroom. His peers also read with him during independent reading time and his frequent rest periods, an activity that Arnez enjoyed and strengthened his peer relationships. Finally, the rehabilitation FOR guided the development of an array of school and home accommodations and modifications made to occupations and school tasks.

Compensatory Frame of Reference

A common FOR associated with the rehabilitation FOR is the compensatory FOR, and it is specifically designed to support individuals for whom recovery of function is not expected (Addy, 2006; Pentland et al., 2017). The underlying goal of the compensatory FOR is to increase occupational participation through environmental changes and the use of compensatory techniques, adaptions, and assistive devices and equipment. The compensatory FOR focuses attention on valued occupational roles and strives to design unique resources to enable an individual to participate successfully in those roles.

Given the progressive nature of Arnez's condition, the compensatory FOR was chosen to specifically guide the development of environmental, activity, and occupational adaptations that would preserve his endurance for school participation. First, it was used to facilitate strategies to educate Arnez and his team about his body function and structure and promote their advocacy for his needs in the school and at home. We taught Arnez about what he could expect from his body and how he could use accommodations and modifications to support his needs. In addition, we taught him how to advocate for his needs within the medical community. We collaboratively created a schedule of needed breaks and rests that supported his health management. Second, along with the rehabilitation FOR, the compensatory FOR enabled us to examine his strengths and develop appropriate supports to enable his access and participation in self-care, education, leisure, and rest occupations at school. We established effective seating and mobility systems in the classroom. We discussed emergency evacuation procedures and field trip opportunities and needs with school administrators. We developed alternate learning activities when Arnez was unable to participate. For example, we established a web-based live stream that enabled Arnez to watch the happenings in the classroom when he was out of the classroom on an extended break.

Goals and Interventions

The SCOPE-IT model provides a solidly, client-centered, occupation-based paradigm in which to base intervention for Arnez. The evaluations and outcome measures that are supported by the SCOPE-IT model aid in the analysis and confirmation of Arnez's capacity to successfully participate in activities presented to him throughout his academic day. Additionally, they provide the necessary data to assist in providing a prognosis by which Arnez's short- and long-term goals can be fashioned. A summary of his health management goals and intervention plan is described in Table 7-4. This is beneficial as Arnez negotiates his academic venture and the support provided within the array of programs he may enter varies; therefore, the level of support he may require from occupational therapy is uncertain and should be a robust discussion within the IEP meeting with the team. The SCOPE-IT model's focus on occupational performance, psychological needs, and environmental impacts provides an effective theoretical guide to consider the student's health management needs with the student's academic and occupational strengths and needs.

TABLE 7-4

Arnez's Health Management Goals and Intervention Plan

OCCUPATIONAL COMPONENT	GOAL (PERSON)	ENVIRONMENTAL/ACTIVITY ADAPTATION/MODIFICATION
Social and emotional health promotion and maintenance	Will identify key areas of occupational interest and develop motivation and competence	Engage in exploration of values and interests across all occupational domains. As he gets older, begin to explore postsecondary and vocational interests.
Symptom and condition management	Will identify changes in health condition and symptomatology	Using educative interventions, explore health conditions and health management and advocacy needs.
Communication with the health care system	Will compose and articulate health care needs and requests to health care providers	Promote the development of advocacy for health care needs and provide instruction/intervention in communicating needs to instructional staff.
Medication management	Will demonstrate awareness of medications and medication schedules	Promote independence in medication management and advocacy per developmental levels and age expectations. Visual schedules and electronic applications (apps) may be helpful to support medication/intervention management.
Physical activity	Will complete classroom arrival and dismissal procedures and other self-care physical activities	Promote independence by modifying the environment, promoting correct body mechanics and ergonomic work and workstations, and providing physical assistance as needed.
Nutrition management	Will identify nutritional needs and develop healthy eating choices	Using educative interventions, promote the development of knowledge of healthy eating habits and maintenance of a healthy lifestyle.
Personal care device management	Will independently manage his power wheelchair, hearing aids, and glasses	Build awareness of the proper use and maintenance of functional and adaptive devices. Behavioral interventions may be helpful in ensuring safe and productive use of devices.

Adapted from American Occupational Therapy Association. (2020). Occupational therapy practice framework: Domain and process (4th ed.). *American Journal of Occupational Therapy, 74*(Suppl. 2), 7412410010p1-7412410010p87. https://doi.org/10.5014/ajot.2020.74S2001

CONCLUSION

In summary, health management is an essential area of occupation and one that occupational therapy practitioners, with their unique understanding of the intersecting educational and health-related needs of students, can be essential in addressing in the school environment. The development of healthy behaviors and health maintenance is an important domain of academic success and is particularly important for students with disabilities. We discussed health curricula in public schools, and, through our case study of Arnez, we examined the role of occupational therapy in health promotion; maintenance of healthy behaviors and lifestyle; and education for the management of illness, injury, and disability needs. In the next chapter, we examine other critical areas of occupation—sleep and rest. Like health management, sleep and rest are restorative and support active engagement in other areas of occupation (AOTA, 2020).

REFERENCES

Addy, L. (2006). *Occupational therapy evidence in practice for physical rehabilitation.* Blackwell.

American Occupational Therapy Association. (2015). *Occupational therapy's role with health promotion.* American Occupational Therapy Association fact sheet. https://irp.cdn-website.com/de1c86c3/files/uploaded/Health%20promotion%20fact%20sheet.pdf

American Occupational Therapy Association. (2020). Occupational therapy practice framework: Domain and process (4th ed.). *American Journal of Occupational Therapy, 74*(Suppl. 2), 7412410010p1-7412410010p87. https://doi.org/10.5014/ajot.2020.74S2001

Bastian, D., Kinney, T., & Garza, A. (2014). *Explore personal care.* Attainment Company.

Centers for Disease Control and Prevention. (2019). National Health Education Standards. https://www.cdc.gov/healthyschools/sher/standards/index.htm

Centers for Disease Control and Prevention. (2022a). Hand hygiene in school and early care and education. https://www.cdc.gov/handwashing/handwashing-school.html

Centers for Disease Control and Prevention. (2022b). Whole School, Whole Community, Whole Child (WSCC). https://www.cdc.gov/healthyschools/wscc/index.htm

Gillen, G. (2014). Occupational therapy interventions for individuals. In B. A. B. Schell, G. Gillen, M. E. Scaffa, & E. S. Cohn (Eds.), *Willard and Spackman's occupational therapy* (12th ed., pp. 322-341). Wolters Kluwer Health/Lippincott Williams & Wilkins.

Haertl, K. H. (2010). The occupational frame of reference: Applying the SCOPE-IT model. In P. Kramer & J. Hinojosa (Eds.), *Frames of Reference for Pediatric Practice.* Lippincott Williams & Wilkins.

Hemmingsson, H., Egilson, S., Hoffman, O., & Kielhofner, G. (2005). The School Setting Interview (SSI) version 3.0. https://moho-irm.uic.edu/productDetails.aspx?aid=10

Heritage Foundation. (2022). School safety initiative. https://www.heritage.org/school-safety

Ikiugu, M. N., Smallfield, S., & Condit, C. (2009). A framework for combining theoretical conceptual practice models in occupational therapy practice. *Canadian Journal of Occupational Therapy, 76*(3), 162-170. https://doi.org/10.1177/000841740907600305

Miller, L. J., Oakland, T., & Herzberg, D. S. (2013). *Goal-Oriented Assessment of Life Skills (GOAL).* WPS.

National Education Association. (2021). Ensuring safe and just schools: Good hygienic practices. https://www.nea.org/professional-excellence/student-engagement/tools-tips/ensuring-safe-and-just-schools-good-hygienic

National Institute of Justice. (2018). NIJ's comprehensive school safety initiative. https://nij.ojp.gov/topics/articles/nijs-comprehensive-school-safety-initiative

Pentland, D., Kantartzis, S., Clausen, M. G., & Witemyer, K. (2017). Occupational therapy and complexity: Defining and describing practice. Royal College of Occupational Therapists. https://www.rcot.co.uk/sites/default/files/OT%20and%20complexity.pdf

Poulsen, A. (2011). Scope-it model: Synthesis of Child, Occupational Performance and Environment In Time. https://www.researchgate.net/publication/43523905_SCOPEIT_Model_Synthesis_of_Child_Occupational_Performance_and_Environment_In_Time/link/53deaeac0cf216e4210c55c2/download

Poulsen, A., Rodger, S., & Ziviani, J. (2006). Understanding children's motivation from a self-determination theoretical perspective: Implications for practice. *Australian Occupational Therapy Journal, 53*(2), 78-86.

Poulsen, A. A., & Ziviani, J. M. (2004). Health enhancing physical activity: Factors influencing engagement patterns in children. *Australian Occupational Therapy Journal, 51*, 69-79.

SchoolSafety. (2022). About SchoolSafety.gov. https://www.schoolsafety.gov/about

U.S. Department of Education Office of Elementary and Secondary Education. (2022). Safe and supportive schools. https://oese.ed.gov/offices/office-of-formula-grants/safe-supportive-schools/

Wrobel, M. J. (2003). *Taking care of myself: A hygiene, puberty and personal curriculum for young people with autism.* Future Horizons.

Ziviani, J., & Poulsen, A. (2017). Synthesis of Child, Occupational, Performance, and Environmental-In Time: A motivational perspective on occupational performance. In J. Hinojosa, P. Kramer, & C. B. Royeen (Eds.), *Perspectives on human occupation—Theories underlying practice.* F. A. Davis.

Rest and Sleep

Caitlin Stanford, OTD, OTR/L

Chapter Objectives

1. Define the occupations of rest and sleep and describe the ways in which they support engagement in other school-related occupations.
2. Identify the ways in which the occupations of rest and sleep support students' active and productive engagement in occupations and activities in the home, school, and community.
3. Describe the ways in which occupational therapy practitioners evaluate and establish theoretically based intervention plans for students with needs in the areas of rest and sleep.

When considering occupations of school-age children, they often are thought of as dynamic, lively, social, and interactive. For example, everyday occupations might include playing with friends, socializing over the lunch table, and actively learning in a vibrant classroom setting. However, for students to fully engage in these energetic activities, they need to participate equally, if not more often, in the restorative occupations of rest and sleep. Rest and sleep are presented together in the fourth edition of the *Occupational Therapy Practice Framework: Domain and Process* (*OTPF-4*; American Occupational Therapy Association [AOTA], 2020), although they are separate occupations each with their own distinct benefit and value. In the *OTPF-4*, rest refers to identifying and engaging in calm, quiet, and relaxing actions that reduce physical and mental activity and restore energy, interest, and

Laverdure, P., & Seruya, F. M. *Theory in School-Based Occupational Therapy Practice: A Practical Application* (pp. 101-117).
DOI: 10.4324/9781003526773-8

TABLE 8-1
Guided Visualization Illustrating the Variables Associated With Sleep
PICTURE THIS ...
Close your eyes. Visualize a perfect night's sleep. What does your room look like; is it dark or slightly lit? What does your bed feel like; are the sheets cool? Flannel? Do you use two pillows and many blankets or one pillow and a sheet? Do you experience nightmares? Do you share the bed with a partner or a pet? Is there noise from outside, a fan, or a sound machine? Now imagine your bedroom as a child; how much control did you have over the amount of light, the bedsheets, the noise, or siblings sleeping next door? Did you share a room? Were you afraid of the dark? Think about the variables that occur while we are sleeping. Some we have a lot of control over. Other factors are harder for us to adjust and affect quality and quantity of sleep daily.

ability to participate in other occupations (AOTA, 2020). Sleep encompasses both sleep preparation, or the routines that enable an individual to prepare for comfortable sleep, and sleep participation, or the participation in sleep activities for oneself and/or others.

REST AND SLEEP OCCUPATIONS

Activities of rest are identified as periods of engagement in "relaxing or other endeavors that restore energy and calm and renew interest in engagement" (AOTA, 2020, p. 32). Examples of rest might include a child coloring by themselves, lying in bed to read a book, or simply sitting and observing others play. Sleep, according to the practice framework (AOTA, 2020), consists of both a sleep preparation phase and active engagement in sleeping. Preparation is defined as activities that settle oneself for sleeping, including habits and routines commonly engaged in before bedtime, such as taking a bath, brushing teeth, or reading a story. Preparatory activities that might occur before a child lays down to close their eyes are typically the observable behaviors associated with sleep and those more commonly addressed by occupational therapy practitioners. Once a child is asleep, the unconscious mind is in control, and the misperception is that occupational engagement halts. One could argue how can you measure the "doing" of sleep if there is no conscious participation (Leive & Morrison, 2020). However, the *OTPF-4* acknowledges the "active engagement" that transpires when the body is at rest for the purpose of sleeping (AOTA, 2020, p. 33).

Active engagement includes many complex components. The breakdown of sleep participation incorporates managing a restful night for a continuous period, navigating overnight toileting and/or hydration when necessary, and sleeping successfully despite environmental and family or social contexts. Using this occupation-based description allows practitioners to understand, assess, and intervene in the processes that organize sleep and critically evaluate the systems that support or negatively impact effective sleep practices (Leive & Morrison, 2020). Particularly for school-age children, there may be factors that obstruct or promote healthy sleep that are out of their control.

Consider the 7-year-old child who shares a bedroom with a 4-year-old sibling or the 10-year-old child living in an urban environment with traffic noise. Table 8-1 explores sleep variables in depth. Also, some early school-age children are reported to cosleep or bed-share with caregivers, rendering sleep a co-occupation. Unwinding to settle into sleep is only the beginning. Sleep remains a basic need for all individuals regardless of age (Leive & Morrison, 2020). As such, the remainder of this chapter primarily focuses on sleep practices and performance. Table 8-2 provides a list of recommended sleep amounts for children from birth to 17 years of age.

TABLE 8-2

Recommended Sleep Amounts in Hours

AGE	RECOMMENDED SLEEP AMOUNTS
Newborn (0 to 3 months)	14 to 17
Infant (4 to 11 months)	12 to 15
Toddler (1 to 2 years)	11 to 14
Preschooler (3 to 5 years)	10 to 13
School-age (6 to 13 years)	9 to 11
Teenager (4 to 17 years)	8 to 10

Data Source: Hirshkowitz, M., Whiton, K., Albert, S. M., Alessi, C., Bruni, O., DonCarlos, L., Hazen, N., Herman, J., Katz, E. S., Kheirandish-Gozal, L., Neubauer, D. N., O'Donnell, A. E., Ohayon, M., Peever, J., Rawding, R., Sachdeva, R. C., Setters, B., Vitiello, M. V., Ware, J. C., & Adams Hillard, P. J. (2015). National Sleep Foundation's sleep time duration recommendations: Methodology and results summary. *Sleep Health, 1*(1), 40-43. https://doi.org/10.1016/j.sleh.2014.12.010

REST AND SLEEP OCCUPATIONS IN SCHOOL

Considering the recommended sleep amounts for a typically developing child, a child spends more time sleeping than engaging in any other occupation. If one were to add up the hours that an individual spends sleeping over a lifetime, it would amount to about one third of their life span (Gupta et al., 2016). It could be assumed then that sleep is a primary occupation. How then, if sleep occurs in the context of the home environment, can school-based occupational therapy practitioners include this primary occupation in the context of school-based practice?

Between 11% and 37% of typically developing school-age children suffer from a sleep disorder (Spira, 2021). That percentage increases to range from 40% to 80% when the child has a special needs diagnosis (Spira, 2021). This makes sleep especially important for school-based occupational therapy practitioners to address because caseloads include students with diagnosed special needs. For an occupational therapy practitioner to ascertain information regarding a child's sleep habits, the first step in the school setting is to conduct an occupational profile to determine how the child is functioning in aspects of the school day. By using an occupational profile, an occupational therapy practitioner can begin to narrow down the performance deficits that may be reported by teachers and students themselves. Additionally, performance factors (e.g., habits, routines) and performance skills (e.g., pacing, initiating, organizing) are impacted and thus measurable within the school context. Research shows the impacts of poor quality and quantity of sleep on school performance include the following (Muratori et al., 2019; Rey et al., 2020):

- Decreased attention to tasks
- Decreased executive functioning skills
- Increased impulsivity
- Decreased mental health including mood, frustration tolerance, and increased aggression
- Negatively impacted social skills

For children who are diagnosed with a disability, the cumulative impacts of a poor night's sleep may lead to the impacts described earlier with the following accompanying concerns (MacDuffie et al., 2020):

- Exacerbation of disability symptoms
- Increase in behavioral issues, such as outbursts
- Increase in restricted and repetitive behaviors

Unlike adults, children who experience sleepiness do not always appear tired. Children may demonstrate sleepy cues such as yawning, fidgeting, and verbalizing "I'm tired" or have dark eyes or circles under the eyes; however, it is far more common for them to demonstrate behaviors that mimic those present in attention-deficit disorder or attention-deficit/hyperactivity disorder. Furthermore, young children do not always have the language or the self-awareness to communicate "tired" or "sleepy" to adults (Owens, Spirito, McGuinn, & Nobile, 2000). Specific to the classroom setting, students who are tired may get out of their seat frequently, have difficulty regulating mood, and display signs of anxiety (Ludwig et al., 2019). The academic implications for a child presenting with poor sleep are an indirect result of the observable behaviors associated with an overtired student.

Poor sleep negatively influences a student's achievement of curricular goals, including the Common Core State Standards in education. The standard areas that apply at the elementary school level include reading, writing, speaking and listening, language, and math. Students who present with decreased attention to task and increased impulsivity are more likely to struggle with reading standard components such as retelling stories, including key details, and actively engaging in reading activities. In an area specific to writing, students struggling with impulsivity along with decreased executive functioning skills may be unable to produce a sequenced, organized writing sample (National Governors Association [NGA] Center for Best Practices, 2010).

As writing standards increase for third, fourth, and fifth grade students, the expectation is that stamina for writing also increases. Specifically, students are expected to "Write routinely over extended time frames (time for research, reflection, and revision) and shorter time frames (a single sitting or a day or two) for a range of discipline-specific tasks, purposes, and audiences" (NGA, 2010) once they begin third grade. Students who struggle to stay seated and alert in class would be unable to meet this standard, thus providing an inaccurate look at true academic ability. Reading standards benefit from the application of social-emotional strategies, in particular "Describe how characters in a story respond to major events and challenges" (NGA, 2010). A sleepy student prone to moodiness and demonstrating poor social skills may not have the awareness to identify emotions in others, particularly characters in writing. Moreover, they may struggle to clearly articulate their thoughts and ideas in both written and oral forms. Relative to the math Common Core State Standards, there is a researched link between math skills and executive functioning skills (Hawes et al., 2019). Any number of the math standards would be negatively influenced by a lack of executive functioning skills secondary to a lack of sleep.

Despite the misperception that sleep is an occupation not applicable to the school setting, there are discernible behaviors resulting from poor sleep that directly correlate to potential areas of academic decline. To better understand how occupational therapy practitioners can address sleep and therefore academic and functional impacts within the school setting, consider the following case.

CASE STUDY

Austin is a 5-year-old boy who is diagnosed with autism spectrum disorder (ASD). In September, he began kindergarten in a coteaching classroom (one general education and one special education teacher) with a one-on-one paraprofessional aide for nonacademic times such as recess, specials, and getting on and off the bus. Austin is seen by the elementary school occupational therapy practitioners for sensory needs and fine motor skills one time per week in a group setting in the therapy room and one time per week in the classroom setting. Austin is typically an outgoing and well-liked student. He likes to engage with peers at his classroom table and has had a few playdates with friends since starting the year.

In November, Austin's coteachers begin to document a change in his behavior. They note that he is distancing himself from peers and does not engage in conversation without increased prompting. He seems irritable and bothered by noises during indoor recess, music class, or smart board video clips. Austin is having a hard time focusing in academic and nonacademic periods and is requiring more input during occupational therapy sessions to help calm his body for working. Additionally, his teachers state that he is struggling to keep up with writing tasks in the classroom. The aide has noted that in the mornings off the bus Austin appears more energetic and engaged, but this quickly fades by specials, when she sees him next. The teachers note the same type of energy increase after lunch, which is evidenced by Austin's demeanor in the afternoon. At conference time, Austin's parents discuss his progress with his teachers and the occupational therapy practitioner. They express observations that Austin is hyperaroused after school (i.e., "bouncing off the walls") and difficult to manage because of his energy. By dinnertime, they report a "crash" in energy level when Austin exhibits outbursts of tears or anger and is very hard to settle. The occupational therapy practitioner begins to see a pattern of decreased focus, an increase in sensory seeking, spikes in energy, and a dip in self-regulation. The occupational therapy practitioner asks probing questions about the rest of the evening, and his mother reports that Austin, who is usually a good sleeper, has begun waking throughout the night. This is exacerbated by bedtime resistance accompanied by his outburst behavior.

A thorough discussion reveals that Austin's sleep preparation can take up to 2 hours, and he is beginning to wake up two to three times each night, sometimes getting out of bed. He needs frequent redirection to stop playing, reading, or watching his tablet before finally settling back to bed. The occupational therapy practitioner feels confident that Austin's changing needs in the classroom are a result of poor sleep but needs to explore this hypothesis in depth. By using an occupational profile (Table 8-3), Austin's occupational therapy practitioner has guiding questions to direct the focus of their investigation into Austin's school performance and how sleep may be affecting academic, social, and emotional participation.

Organizing Model of Practice: Canadian Model of Occupational Performance and Engagement

Occupational therapy practitioners working in school settings lack a straightforward framework that allows them to integrate sleep into practice. Thus, the concept of an organizing model of practice is crucial to help guide occupational therapy practitioners through the occupational therapy process from evaluation to outcomes (Ikiugu & Smallfield, 2011). To address Austin's challenges, we chose the Canadian Model of Occupational Performance and Engagement (CMOP-E; Enemark Larsen et al., 2020). The CMOP-E focuses on three primary components: person, occupation, and environment. The guiding principles of this model are enablement of occupation and client centeredness. The person component is illustrated as having spirituality at the core with affective (feeling), physical (doing), and cognitive (thinking) capabilities. Occupation encompasses areas of productivity, self-care, and leisure. Lastly, environment takes into consideration the contexts of physical, institutional, cultural, and social (Polatajko et al., 2007). Furthermore, the CMOP-E takes the relationship one step further. Engagement (E) is added to stress that not only does the person-occupation-environment triad combine for optimal functional performance but also merges for full occupational engagement. The concept of engagement elevates the CMOP-E by suggesting that merely participating in an occupation does not fulfill the occupation prong. Engagement implies a higher-level participation

TABLE 8-3

Austin's Occupational Profile

What concerns do Austin and his team have about his occupational engagement?	Decrease in social interactions Decrease in attention to task Increase in irritability Change in ability to self-regulate Difficulty with writing tasks
In what occupations is Austin successful, and what barriers impact his success?	Austin is successful in morning routine tasks (getting off the bus, unpacking). Generally, Austin does well with behavior and academics; he is a rule follower, motivated to do well, and is a strong reader with the ability to complete high-level math concepts. Barriers reported are his irritability and increased mood changes. Barriers include that Austin's performance varies throughout the day depending on the time. Austin is struggling to carry over strategies from occupational therapy into the classroom for writing tasks.
What is Austin's occupational history?	Austin is a 5-year-old kindergarten student. He attends a full-day inclusive classroom setting with access to a personal aide for nonacademic times. He currently attends occupational therapy for sensory needs and fine motor skills, including self-regulatory strategies and handwriting. Aside from school, Austin reports an interest in dinosaurs, enjoys math, and has a strong relationship with his family.
What are Austin's and his team's personal interests and values?	Austin values his friendships and has a strong interest in doing well in school. His teachers report wanting to see Austin re-engage in the social relationships he has made. His parents value a calm, peaceful end to the day and are invested in helping Austin sleep through the night.

(continued)

TABLE 8-3 (CONTINUED)
Austin's Occupational Profile

What aspects of the contexts do Austin and his team see as supporting engagement in desired occupations, and what aspects are inhibiting engagement?

	SUPPORTING	INHIBITING
ENVIRONMENT	Access to a general and special education teacher in school	Time of day impacts behavior, mood, and ability.
PERSONAL	Austin has made friends in the classroom. Austin has strong family relationships, and his parents are supportive and willing to work with his team in school. Austin is verbal. Austin does well with rules and clear expectations.	Increased irritability impacts Austin's ability to appropriately interact with his friends and peers. Difficulty with handwriting tasks may begin to lead to a lack of self-esteem and frustration, further exacerbating the irritability. Although verbal, Austin is unable to connect identified emotions to context.
PERFORMANCE PATTERNS	Consistent school routines give Austin structure and clear expectations for success. Austin's role as a student means access to supports in school such as occupational therapy and a personal aide.	Austin's bedtime routine is working against his needs and impacts his quality and quantity of sleep. The structured school day does not allow for flexibility in habits and routines. Austin can hyperfocus on tasks, impacting his ability to move from activity to activity.

What client factors do Austin and his team see as supporting engagement in desired occupations, and what aspects are inhibiting engagement?

	SUPPORTING	INHIBITING
VALUES, BELIEFS, AND SPIRITUALITY	Austin's team feels strongly that he can implement strategies independently with guidance from his paraprofessional. The team values a collaborative effort with the family and is open to working on sleep goals in the school environment.	Austin is starting to express frustration over his handwriting, believing this makes him less capable. The team must consider the school environment first, which may impact the occupational therapy practitioner's ability to support the family at times.
BODY FUNCTIONS	Bursts of energy allow Austin to engage in morning tasks and work after lunch.	Lack of sleep is impacting Austin's self-regulation and mood.
BODY STRUCTURES	Austin's body structures are reported and observed to be intact.	Austin's physical skills are reported to be of no concern based on intact body structures.

(continued)

TABLE 8-3 (CONTINUED)	
Austin's Occupational Profile	
What are Austin's and his team's priorities and desired goals?	
OCCUPATIONAL PERFORMANCE	To increase self-regulatory skills within the classroom To increase participation and social skills To increase carryover and skill in handwriting, improving Austin's ability to perform as a student
PREVENTION	To provide education to Austin, his team, and his parents on healthy sleep habits as well as bedtime routine strategies to prevent sleep loss and fatigue in school
HEALTH AND WELLNESS	To improve overall sleep functions in the home as well as improve mood and attention and decrease irritability in the classroom setting
QUALITY OF LIFE AND WELL-BEING	To provide Austin with the language and strategies for healthy sleep tactics as they apply to school and home to increase independence, self-awareness, and self-confidence
PARTICIPATION AND ROLE COMPETENCE	To increase Austin's engagement with his peers by addressing his self-regulation and mood To assist Austin in meeting the fine motor and handwriting demands of the classroom
OCCUPATIONAL JUSTICE	To ensure that Austin is successful in maintaining his friendships despite difficulty with his mood and social engagement To offer opportunities for Austin to focus on his self-regulatory needs while also ensuring he can maintain the appropriate classroom demands

Adapted from American Occupational Therapy Association. (2020). AOTA occupational profile template. https://www.aota.org/-/media/Corporate/Files/Practice/Manage/Documentation/AOTA-Occupational-Profile-Template.pdf

concept when performance has personal meaning and relates to a social role (Enemark Larsen et al., 2020). Thus, the CMOP-E proposes that engagement and participation are different modes of occupation that are similarly defined but separate concepts.

The CMOP-E is well suited as a guiding model of practice to address sleep in school practice. The concept of person is straightforward in that a school-based occupational therapy practitioner should consider negative impacts that poor sleep has on areas of affect, cognition, and performance skills. Examples may include supporting a student's ability to regulate mood when overtired or working with teachers to identify the subtle differences between sleep-related attention deficits and biological attention deficits. Relative to occupation, sleep falls under the category of self-care and overlaps with leisure if an occupational therapy practitioner includes the preferred habits and routines necessary for rest and unwinding before sleeping. Productivity can be measured by quantifying school performance, closing the circle on occupation. Therefore, the application of theory to address personal contexts and occupational capabilities regarding sleep can be seamlessly included in current school-based evaluation, intervention, and outcome processes.

What sets the CMOP-E apart from other applicable models is the environmental contexts and the engagement factor. Both dynamic concepts serve as essential framework pieces that assist school-based occupational therapy practitioners in making an argument for addressing sleep within the context of the school system. Because direct observation of quantity and quality of sleep does not happen within the school context, it is difficult for occupational therapy practitioners to address the environment relative to the physical context. However, school-based occupational therapy practitioners can address the environment through the concepts of institution, culture, and society. For example, at an institutional level, occupational therapy practitioners can explore how the school supports students when they arrive to class after a difficult night's sleep or how staff encourages self-care and teaches healthy sleep habits to students who are cognitively able to carry over skills to the home setting. Furthermore, occupational therapy practitioners can address the cultural and societal expectations of sleep through administrator or parent/caregiver education and training. Educating team members on recommended sleep amounts or participating in discussions regarding school start and end times are ways to advocate in a larger context. This also includes being informed and informing others of possible cultural sleep differences, such as cosleeping.

Looking at engagement allows school-based occupational therapy practitioners to stretch beyond the limits of academic performance and assess how invested a student is in a preferred school-based occupation. For example, a student may continue to ride the bus, unpack in the classroom, and initiate morning work but lack the thoughtfulness that engagement suggests, thereby demonstrating decreased performance while still participating. This lack of engagement can be an informative observation that occupational therapy practitioners might miss given a hectic school schedule. Having teachers, student support staff, and parents report on student engagement in multiple areas is an effective way to measure the E in CMOP-E theory.

If the CMOP-E provides a guiding framework, how then can it be specifically applied to the evaluation process of sleep in the school setting? Completing a detailed occupational profile as a first step assists an occupational therapy practitioner in evaluating and choosing the most appropriate assessments given the student's needs. An occupational therapy practitioner must be familiar with sleep assessments that apply in the context of the school system. Table 8-4 provides a brief list of applicable sleep assessments.

After considering relevant information, Austin's occupational therapy practitioner determines that although Austin's sleep at home is crucial to his school performance, the primary context impacted is the classroom setting and academic tasks. Austin's occupational therapy practitioner cannot justify addressing at-home needs through assessment data; they can only support Austin at home through indirect means. The occupational therapy practitioner also concludes that in keeping with the principle of engagement, Austin's input to the evaluation is valuable. To ensure a strong client-centered approach, the evaluation should take into consideration what preferred tasks are negatively impacted by poor engagement. Using an occupation-based approach to evaluation and considering the components of the CMOP-E that Austin's occupational therapy practitioner would want to explore, a reasonable assumption is to use sleep assessments that target child self-report and teacher report. Additionally, a functional, holistic look at occupational performance to better understand participation and engagement is essential.

After completing an evaluation that consists of relevant sleep assessments and a holistic assessment aimed at occupational participation, Austin's areas of strength are as follows:

- Austin can, with prompting, verbalize that he is "grouchy" and "annoyed" during the day.
- His teachers and aide report he interacts with peers with less prompting during lunch and specials (except music).
- Austin reports enjoying school and is observed to be a rule follower; once he knows the expectations, he is motivated to achieve them.
- Austin is a bright child. Despite fine motor challenges, he can complete math concepts at a high level and can read beyond a kindergarten level.

TABLE 8-4

Applicable Sleep Assessments

SLEEP ASSESSMENT	DESCRIPTION
BEARS Sleep Screening Tool	B (bedtime problems), E (excessive sleepiness), A (awakening during the night), R (regularity of evening sleep times and morning awakenings), and S (sleep-related breathing problems or snoring).
	Nonstandardized screener for children 2 to 18 years old. Used to determine if further sleep evaluations/referrals are necessary (Owens & Dalzell, 2005).
Family Inventory of Sleep Habits	Family Inventory of Sleep Habits specifically measures sleep in children with ASD ages 3 to 10 years. Reliable and valid; looks at daytime/prebed habits, bedtime routine, and sleep environment (Malow et al., 2009).
Sleep Self-Report Questionnaire	Sleep Self-Report Questionnaire is a child report given in schools to children ages 7 to 12 years old. Multidimensional assessing sleep duration, night waking, and daytime sleepiness. Likert scale 26-item short checklist; correlated with domains of the Children's Sleep Habits Questionnaire (CSHQ; Owens, Spirito, McGuinn, & Nobile, 2000).
Teacher's Daytime Sleepiness Questionnaire	Teacher's Daytime Sleepiness Questionnaire looks at classroom concerns that may be a result of poor sleep such as napping, yawning, aggression, and hyperactivity. It takes 3 to 5 minutes to be completed and consists of Likert scale questions; it is for children 4 to 10 years old. Higher scores indicate the presence of sleep problems (Owens, Spirito, McGuinn, & Nobile, 2000).
CSHQ	CSHQ is a well-established valid screener for children ages 4 to 10 years. Parent report of 35 items (8 subtests). Screens for both behavioral and medical sleep concerns, including parasomnias and sleep-disordered breathing. Research suggests it is well applied to populations with ASD (Katz et al., 2018; Owens, Spirito, & McGuinn, 2000).

Austin's areas of challenge are as follows:

- Austin appears apathetic in the classroom; he prefers his teachers and aide to tell him what to do and will ask clarifying questions before attempting work independently.
- Austin is struggling to keep up with handwriting demands in the classroom; he is unable to effectively carry over strategies from occupational therapy sessions.
- He shows signs of decreased self-regulation and periods of sensory-seeking and sensory-avoiding behaviors.
- Austin is unable to articulate why he is "grouchy" and "annoyed." He is unable to connect his poor sleep at home with his feelings at school.
- Once Austin feels comfortable with a task, he often hyperfocuses on completion and struggles to take a break from working once engaged.

Complementary Models of Practice

The CMOP-E is an appropriate model to address participation and engagement secondary to the concerns regarding Austin's inability to initiate on his own; poor connections between the affective, physical, and cognitive aspects of the person; and his inability to appropriately disengage from a task. However, as we continue to discuss in this chapter, completing the evaluation process and providing interventions for and measuring outcomes of sleep-related goals are complex and dynamic tasks. A closer analysis of Austin's case indicates there remains a need to tie in complementary models of practice to effectively target all of Austin's areas of functioning (Ikiugu & Smallfield, 2011). Based on the occupational profile and assessments, the two complementary models that are most appropriate are sensory integration and a behavioral approach.

Dunn's Model of Sensory Processing

To address the unique neurologic processes that organize sensory input from the environment and within the body to produce an effective and appropriate response, Winnie Dunn's Model of Sensory Processing was chosen as the focus for Austin's case because the language developed to describe sensory needs fits Austin's particular patterns of sensory regulation and dysregulation. Additionally, research suggests that Dunn's model and subsequent assessments are applicable to sleep as a concern for children with ASD (Tzischinsky et al., 2018). Dunn (2007) proposes that responses to sensory stimuli occur in four categories, each resulting from the intersection of a person's neurologic threshold with their self-regulation.

The neurologic threshold refers to the point at which a person takes in enough sensory stimuli such that it elicits a response from the body. Self-regulation is defined as the individual's ability to engage in passive or active responses to the sensory input provided (Dunn, 2007; Metz et al., 2019). The four categories Dunn (2007) proposes to describe sensory processing are sensory seeking, sensory avoiding, sensory sensitivity, and low regulation. Each of these constructs falls on a continuum, and individuals may fall into different categories for different sensory stimuli. Sensory-seeking individuals demonstrate a high threshold, needing very little stimuli to trigger a response, and active self-regulation, meaning they actively engage in a behavioral response to respond to the stimuli. Sensory-avoiding individuals demonstrate a low threshold and active self-regulation (Dunn, 2007). Children in the sensory-sensitivity category demonstrate low thresholds with passive regulation. The final category, low registration, indicates a child with a low threshold and passive response strategies (Dunn, 2007). Low-registration children may require increased stimuli and support to respond appropriately.

If children demonstrate low sensory thresholds, they may be quick to notice and respond to stimuli because their systems are easily activated (Metz et al., 2019). This can result in negative behavioral responses in an effort to mitigate the incoming stimuli. Children who demonstrate high sensory thresholds to stimuli may be less responsive, thereby missing sensory information that others respond to (Metz et al., 2019). This type of response may result in children failing to react appropriately to sensory input, including a delayed reaction or no reaction at all. Austin's occupational therapy practitioner can use Dunn's proposed theoretical constructs and supplemental assessments to further understand Austin's sensory processing throughout the day. By understanding which category Austin falls into and when the behavioral response is maladaptive to functioning, the occupational therapy practitioner can better address Austin's sensory needs for classroom success.

Using Dunn's model as a complement to the CMOP-E has benefits in addressing the occupation of sleep because sensory processing has a relationship with both sleep and the concept of engagement. Research suggests a correlation between sensory processing difficulties, particularly tactile sensitivity, and sleep concerns in typically developing children (Spira, 2021). Studies indicate that the link between sensory processing and sleep concerns is more likely when comorbid with impending conditions such as ASD; hyperarousal in children experiencing neurologic conditions may be a factor (Spira, 2021). Up to 80% of children with ASD are likely to have disturbed sleep, leading to an increase in the severity of their ASD symptoms and self-injurious behaviors and a decrease in cognitive or emotional functioning (Waddington et al., 2020). These correlations suggest that it is difficult to separate sleep concerns from sensory functioning in both typically and atypically developing students, thereby strengthening the argument for use of the sensory processing approach.

Behavior Frame of Reference

The second complementary approach, a behavioral model, is an effective partner to the CMOP-E and Dunn's models to support a measurable and data-driven method to interventions. More specifically, the behavioral frame of reference, which focuses on behavior modifications and shaping behavior using applied strategies (Cho, 2022), can be effective in addressing sleep (Mindell et al., 2006) and is a particularly effective approach to use with children diagnosed with ASD (Case-Smith & Arbesman, 2008; Mindell et al., 2006). Strategies used under the behavioral frame of reference include the use of a token economy system, reinforcement, systematic desensitization, and extinction (Cho, 2022). Not all strategies are applicable to all behaviors; however, a critical component of a behavioral approach is to complete a functional analysis of the problem behaviors and ascertain the antecedents to the behavior (Case-Smith & Arbesman, 2008).

Once the problem behaviors have been identified, a token economy can be established to support positive reinforcement of a desired behavioral outcome. A token economy system describes the use of positive reinforcement (typically a reward) in exchange for the completion of a desired task or behavior (Bourne, 2018). Research demonstrates that a token economy system is effective for improving behaviors and is increasingly more effective when combined with a self-monitoring aspect; task completion behaviors are a primary target for token economy systems (Bourne, 2018). Behavioral modifications are an appropriate choice within the school system in that this approach includes the collection of baseline and progress data (Cho, 2022). It may be difficult for an occupational therapy practitioner to advocate why there is a need to address sleep in the academic setting; collecting measurable data that demonstrate the effectiveness of an intervention can be key to administrative support. Furthermore, behavioral approaches to sleep intervention are often found to be more acceptable to parents and children, avoid pharmaceutical methods that may lead to side effects, and have greater potential to generalize to daytime concerns (Mindell et al., 2006). This makes behavioral modification an ideal choice in Austin's case because the occupational therapy practitioner may use similar strategies in the classroom and home setting, thereby increasing carryover.

In Austin's case, his parents report maladaptive behaviors (reading and using a tablet) are exacerbating Austin's night waking, thereby impacting sleep quantity. This suggests that Austin has poor sleep hygiene, which can be defined as behavioral and environmental modifications that provide the foundation for healthy sleep (Rottapel et al., 2020). To positively influence Austin's sleep behaviors through the school system, the occupational therapy practitioner can consider educating Austin on sleep hygiene and instructing Austin and his parents on how to use a token economy to promote the individual sleep habits that make up sleep hygiene. Education of healthy sleep hygiene can be incorporated in Austin's typical occupational therapy session. The occupational therapy practitioner can work with Austin to discuss the habits and routines that fit best at home and then use a gross motor game while asking Austin to repeat each habit during a specific game movement. Austin can work toward handwriting goals by copying portions or a modified list of these same habits. The occupational therapy practitioner may also work on education during a traditional therapy session incorporating fine motor skills, sequencing, and handwriting by having Austin create his own healthy sleep habit checklist for the home environment. Education of the parent can be delivered via phone call, at a parent–teacher conference, at an Individualized Education Program meeting, or with parent participation at Austin's individual session to understand healthy sleep habits. Table 8-5 provides a brief list of healthy sleep habit examples.

TABLE 8-5

Sleep Hygiene: Healthy Sleep Habit Examples

- Removing small screens from the sleep space (Dube et al., 2017)
- Creating a bedtime routine consisting of consistent, predictable steps (Mindell & Williamson, 2018)
- Restricting bedtime routines to under 40 minutes (Mindell & Williamson, 2018)
- Maintain consistent bed and wake time (no more than 60 minutes of variations in daily schedules; Allen et al., 2016)
- Modify daytime activities such as eating and physical activity to a schedule that positively promotes sleep (Suni, 2022)
- Modify the bedroom environment for comfort; dim lights, use music or scents, reduce noise (Suni, 2022)

As mentioned previously, behavioral strategies may be generalized to target task completion (Mindell et al., 2006) in the academic setting and used to positively reinforce rest and sensory-based breaks throughout the day. For example, the occupational therapy practitioner works with Austin and his teacher to target Austin's hyperfocus, which inhibits his ability to disengage and rest in the classroom. The occupational therapy practitioner then encourages Austin to choose a preferential activity to earn as a reward for the behavior of disengaging from a task when prompted. Austin then earns points (or tokens) each time he is able to disengage, thereby earning the preferential activity when he reaches an agreed-on target number of disengagements. Similarly, when Austin independently requests a sensory break or works with the occupational therapy practitioner to successfully use sensory equipment appropriately during a break, Austin may earn tokens toward a preferred reward. Once this strategy has been effective in the classroom setting, the occupational therapy practitioner can discuss with the parents the use of a token system at home to reinforce the previously identified sleep habits.

Goals and Interventions

After analyzing Austin's needs, the overall goal would be for him to increase his sleep quality and quantity. To assist in this goal, the occupational therapy practitioner recognizes that certain factors are beyond school-based control and therefore more difficult to intervene and monitor. The strength of the behavioral approach addresses these concerns with parent education and home carryover. The process then evolves to a focus on factors that support occupational performance in the classroom setting and acknowledge how to creatively promote healthy sleep in the home through caregiver and child support. Using the critical thinking process that allows sleep to be considered under the umbrella of school-based practice, an occupational therapy practitioner can craft school-based, functional, and academically relevant sleep goals; this is why the use of complementary models of practice is emphasized.

Goals cannot be measured without specific data; incorporating components of Dunn's Model of Sensory Processing and a behavioral approach allow the school-based occupational therapy practitioner to create specific, measurable goals that apply to academic areas. This is also a suitable time to reintroduce the concept of rest as it relates to a classroom setting. Rest is an important part of daily living in that it allows an individual to purposefully cease taxing activities to help "restore energy and calm and renew interest in engagement" (AOTA, 2020, p. 32). Providing rest breaks or rest activities to tired students allows them time to disengage in order to then re-engage with vigor. Returning to the case of Austin, the most appropriate start is to provide immediate support when Austin's classroom behaviors indicate too little sleep. Long-term goal areas might include working to self-regulate using sensory-based strategies, increasing self-awareness of and the ability to self-report on sleep, using behavior supports to effectively address rest practices, and working with the teachers and student to educate and advocate for sleep needs.

The following are examples of sleep-related goals:

- Austin will effectively communicate his level of tiredness when asked using a sleep scale (e.g., not sleepy, a little sleepy, a lot sleepy).
- Allow Austin to choose strategies from a predetermined list of sensory-based equipment/activities to aid in attention in the classroom setting.
- Establish routines with Austin and his teachers and aide that allow for rest breaks before or during challenging tasks.
- Austin will successfully identify two healthy sleep habits that promote good sleeping.

The occupational therapy practitioner uses assessment data to establish a baseline of functioning and can repeat the evaluation measures as appropriate to gain insight into progress with sleep goals and academic and functional performance. The occupational therapy practitioner can rely on session and classroom observation as well as informal teacher reports to identify the change in engagement as it applies to occupational participation. Austin's occupational therapy practitioner is looking to address improvement in sensory processing and tolerance of sensory stimuli, address sleep through a broad health and wellness approach, increase participation in the classroom setting through engagement, and assist Austin in effectively meeting the classroom demands. Now that goal areas have been established and an appropriate approach has been chosen, the occupational therapy practitioner can move forward with an intervention plan. An intervention plan must include components such as the approach to intervention, the type of intervention (AOTA, 2020), the service delivery model, and appropriate intervention activities.

The following approaches to intervention were chosen to address his needs:

- Establish/restore: Establish healthy sleep routines in the home setting while adhering to school objectives, restore sensory processing abilities to the previously reported baseline, and establish school routines to allow for rest and sensory breaks.
- Maintain: Communicate with Austin's aide, teachers, and parents to ensure maintenance and carryover of any established skills.
- Modify: Support Austin through the modifications of his school day or academic tasks to allow for independence and success.

Table 8-6 illustrates the types of interventions chosen to address his needs.

To close the loop between theory and intervention, the sample intervention plan can be addressed using a focus on engagement in the classroom through the provision of sensory integration strategies and behavioral supports, such as a reward system, to help motivate Austin to use strategies and engage with purpose. By structuring sleep in the school setting with the CMOP-E theory, a school-based occupational therapy practitioner ensures the inclusion of evidence-based guidance for maximum student success.

TABLE 8-6

Types of Interventions

OCCUPATIONS AND ACTIVITIES	ASSISTIVE TECHNOLOGY AND ENVIRONMENTAL MODIFICATIONS	SELF-REGULATION	EDUCATION AND TRAINING	ADVOCACY
Introduce a sleep scale and use in-session activities to learn appropriate language and self-awareness of sleep level. Use methods such as breaking down of assignments, shortening assignments, and taking breaks in between tasks. Continue to support fine motor goals as necessary through client-centered activities.	Modify schedule to allow for rest break throughout the day. Use meditation or other calming application (apps) to allow for scheduled periods of disengagement. Work with teachers to modify schedules on Monday mornings or after holiday breaks to allow for a slower transition back to class routines. Modify the end of the day schedule to allow for a calming period before getting on the bus.	Provide opportunities for sensory-based strategies to support when overtired. Teach how to use a "toolbox" of strategies to increase self-awareness and self-regulation throughout the day. Provide increased sensory integration activities in sessions to help maintain a regulated state throughout the day to avoid overstimulation at the end of the day.	Train teachers and his aide on Austin's sleep scale. Training Austin and his parents on the use of apps for unwinding and meditation before sleeping. Parental education on healthy sleep environments, sleep routines, and importance of sleep regularity. Education and training of teachers and staff to recognize sleep-related performance deficits.	Work with school administration and teachers to educate on sleep deficits in children and the importance of healthy sleep practices. Advocate at the administrative level to evaluate school start times. Advocate for whole-school healthy sleep initiates with interprofessional teams, such as school counselors, nurses, and psychologists.

CONCLUSION

As discussed in this chapter, rest and sleep are critical occupations to be examined and addressed by occupational therapy practitioners in school practice. We described rest and sleep and their value to students as they learn, play, and interact in home and school. We examined the characteristics of rest and sleep in the developing child and challenges that often occur when rest and sleep are disrupted. Although sleep occurs in the home environment, it is paramount that occupational therapy practitioners address it as a part of their occupational profile and analysis because of its possible influence on regulation, attention, endurance, participation, and learning. In the next chapter, we continue to examine the role of occupational therapy practitioners who use occupation-based theoretical foundations to support the evaluation and intervention planning for students. We also examine education and work, two intersecting occupations that are important to the function and participation of students.

REFERENCES

Allen, S. L., Howlett, M. D., Coulombe, J. A., & Corkum, P. V. (2016). ABCs of SLEEPING: A review of the evidence behind pediatric sleep practice recommendations. *Sleep Medicine Reviews, 29*, 1-14. https://doi.org/10.1016/j.smrv.2015.08.006

American Occupational Therapy Association. (2020). Occupational therapy practice framework: Domain and process (4th ed.). *American Journal of Occupational Therapy, 74*(Suppl. 2), 7412410010p1-7412410010p87. https://doi.org/10.5014/ajot.2020.74S2001

Bourne, P. (2018). A token economy: An approach used for behavior modifications among disruptive primary school children. *MOJ Public Health, 7*(3), 89-99. https://doi.org/10.15406/mojph.2018.07.00212

Case-Smith, J., & Arbesman, M. (2008). Evidence-based review of interventions for autism used in or of relevance to occupational therapy. *American Journal of Occupational Therapy, 62*(4), 416-429.

Cho, M. (2022). *Behavioral frame of reference.* OT theory. https://ottheory.com/therapy-model/behavioral-frame-reference

Dube, N., Khan, K., Loehr, S., Chu, Y., & Veugelers, P. (2017). The use of entertainment and communication technologies before sleep could affect sleep and weight status: A population-based study among children. *International Journal of Behavioral Nutrition and Physical Activity, 14*(1), 1-15. https://doi.org/10.1186/s12966-017-0547-2

Dunn, W. (2007). Supporting children to participate successfully in everyday life by using sensory processing knowledge. *Infants & Young Children, 20*(2), 84-101.

Enemark Larsen, A., Wehberg, S., & Christensen, J. R. (2020). Looking into the content of the Canadian Occupational Performance Measure (COPM): A Danish cross-sectional study. *Occupational Therapy International, 2020,* 9573950-9573950. https://doi.org/10.1155/2020/9573950

Gupta, R., Kandpal, S. D., Goel, D., Mittal, N., Dhyani, M., & Mittal, M. (2016). Sleep-patterns, co-sleeping and parent's perception of sleep among school children: Comparison of domicile and gender. *Sleep Science, 9*(3), 192-197. https://doi.org/10.1016/j.slsci.2016.07.003

Hawes, Z., Moss, J., Caswell, B., Seo, J., & Ansari, D. (2019). Relations between numerical, spatial, and executive function skills and mathematics achievement: A latent-variable approach. *Cognitive Psychology, 109,* 68-90. https://doi.org/10.1016/j.cogpsych.2018.12.002

Ikiugu, M., & Smallfield, S. (2011). Ikiugu's eclectic method of combining theoretical conceptual practice models in occupational therapy. *Australian Occupational Therapy Journal, 58*(6), 437-446. https://doi.org/10.1111/j.1440-1630.2011.00968.x

Katz, T., Shui, A. M., Johnson, C. R., Richdale, A. L., Reynolds, A. M., Scahill, L., & Malow, B. A. (2018). Modification of the children's sleep habits questionnaire for children with autism spectrum disorder. *Journal of Autism and Developmental Disorders, 48*(8), 2629-2641. https://doi.org/10.1007/s10803-018-3520-2

Leive, L., & Morrison, R. (2020). Essential characteristics of sleep from the occupational science perspective. *Cadernos Brasileiros de Terapia Ocupacional, 28*(3), 1072-1092. https://doi.org/10.4322/2526-8910.ctoARF1954

Ludwig, B., Smith, S. S., & Heussler, H. (2019). Exploring the association between perceived excessive daytime sleepiness in children and academic outcomes. *Issues in Educational Research, 29*(3), 841-857.

MacDuffie, K. E., Munson, J., Greenson, J., Ward, T. M., Rogers, S. J., Dawson, G., & Estes, A. (2020). Sleep problems and trajectories of restricted and repetitive behaviors in children with neurodevelopmental disabilities. *Journal of Autism and Developmental Disorders, 50*(11), 3844-3856. https://doi.org/10.1007/s10803-020-04438-y

Malow, B. A., Crowe, C., Henderson, L., McGrew, S. G., Wang, I., Song, Y., & Stone, W. L. (2009). A sleep habits questionnaire for children with autism spectrum disorders. *Journal of Child Neurology, 24*(1), 19-24. https://doi.org/10.177/0883073808321044

Metz, A. E., Boling, D., DeVore, A., Holladay, H., Liao, J. F., & Vlutch, K. V. (2019). Dunn's model of sensory processing: An investigation of the axes of the four-quadrant model in healthy adults. *Brain Sciences, 9*(2), 35-50. https://doi.org/10.3390/brainsci9020035

Mindell, J. A., Kuhn, B., Lewin, D. S., Meltzer, L. J., Sadeh, A. (2006). Behavioral treatment of bedtime problems and night wakings in infants and young children. *Sleep, 29*(10), 1263-1276. https://doi.org/10.1093/sleep/29.10.1263

Mindell, J. A., & Williamson, A. A. (2018). Benefits of a bedtime routine in young children: Sleep, development, and beyond. *Sleep Medicine Reviews, 40*, 93-108. https://doi.org/10.1016/j.smrv.2017.10.007

Muratori, P., Menicucci, D., Lai, E., Battaglia, F., Bontempelli, L., Chericoni, N., & Gemignani, A. (2019). Linking sleep to externalizing behavioral difficulties: A longitudinal psychometric survey in a cohort of Italian school-age children. *The Journal of Primary Prevention, 40*, 231-241. https://doi.org/10.1007/s10935-019-00547-2

National Governors Association Center for Best Practices, Council of Chief State School Officers. (2010). *Common core state standards.* Author. http://corestandards.org/

Owens, J. A., & Dalzell, V. (2005). Use of the 'BEARS' sleep screening tool in a pediatric residents' continuity clinic: A pilot study. *Sleep Medicine, 6*(1), 63-69.

Owens, J. A., Spirito, A., & McGuinn, M. (2000). The Children's Sleep Habits Questionnaire (CSHQ): Psychometric properties of a survey instrument for school-aged children. *Sleep, 23*(8), 1043-1051.

Owens, J. A., Spirito, A., McGuinn, M., & Nobile, C. (2000). Sleep habits and sleep disturbance in elementary school-aged children. *Journal of Developmental and Behavioral Pediatrics, 21*(1), 27-36.

Polatajko, H. J., Townsend, E. A., & Craik, J. (2007). Canadian Model of Occupational Performance and Engagement (CMOP-E). In E. A. Townsend & H. J. Polatajko (Eds.), *Enabling occupation I: Advancing an occupational therapy vision of health, well-being, & justice through occupation* (p. 23). CAOT Publications ACE.

Rey, A. E., Guignard-Perret, A., Imler-Weber, F., Garcia-Larrea, L., & Mazza, S. (2020). Improving sleep, cognitive functioning and academic performance with sleep education at school in children. *Learning and Instruction, 65*, 1-9. https://doi.org/10.1016/j.learninstruc.2019.101270

Rottapel, R. E., Zhou, E. S., Spadola, C. E., Clark, C. R., Kontos, E. Z., Laver, K., Chen, J. T., Redline, S., & Bertisch, S. M. (2020). Adapting sleep hygiene for community interventions: a qualitative investigation of sleep hygiene behaviors among racially/ethnically diverse, low-income adults. *Sleep Health, 6*(2), 205-213. https://doi.org/10.1016/j.sleh.2019.12.009

Spira, G. (2021). A sensory intervention to improve sleep behaviours and sensory processing behaviours of children with sensory processing disorders. *Irish Journal of Occupational Therapy, 49*(1), 11-20. https://doi.org/10.1108/IJOT-09-2020-0014

Suni, E. (2022, September 29). *Sleep hygiene.* Sleep Foundation. https://www.sleepfoundation.org/sleep-hygiene

Tzischinsky, O., Meiri, G., Manelis, L., Bar-Sinai, A., Flusser, H., Michaelovski, A., Zivan, O., Ilan, M., Faroy, M., Menashe, I., & Dinstein, I. (2018). Sleep disturbances are associated with specific sensory sensitivities in children with autism. *Molecular Autism, 9*, 22. https://doi.org/10.1186/s13229-018-0206-8

Waddington, H., McLay, L., & Woods, L. (2020). Child and family characteristics associated with sleep disturbance in children with autism spectrum disorder. *Journal of Autism and Developmental Disorders, 50*(11), 4121-4132. https://doi.org/10.1007/s10803-020-04475-7

9

Education and Work

Mindy Garfinkel, OTD, OTR/L, ATP

Chapter Objectives

1. Define education and work occupations and describe the ways in which these occupations are experienced in school by students.
2. Identify the alignment and guidance of the Individuals with Disabilities Education Act (IDEA), the Every Student Succeeds Act, and the American Occupational Therapy Association's (AOTA's) fourth edition of the *Occupational Therapy Practice Framework: Domain and Process (OTPF-4)* for practice in educational settings.
3. Discuss the use of occupation-based theoretical foundations to support the needs for students with educational disabilities.

The AOTA in the *OTPF-4* defines education as "activities involved in learning and participating in the educational environment" (AOTA, 2020, p. 76). This may include engagement in academic (e.g., learning curriculum), nonacademic (e.g., recess and lunch), extracurricular (e.g., activities occurring outside the school day), technological (e.g., coding and use of tablets), and vocational (i.e., activities designed to prepare a student for work) pursuits or skills (AOTA, 2020). The U.S. Department of Education (DOE) describes the main outcomes of formal education in the public school system as learning and preparation for productivity in the workforce (Cahill & Beisbier, 2020). School-based academic and nonacademic learning opportunities support a student's prevocational and vocational development and a life of productive contribution to society (Cahill & Beisbier, 2020).

Laverdure, P., & Seruya, F. M. *Theory in School-Based Occupational Therapy Practice: A Practical Application* (pp. 119-134).
DOI: 10.4324/9781003526773-9

Work is defined as exertion as it relates to the creation, production, delivery, or management of things or services. The benefits of work may be nonfinancial or financial (Christiansen & Townsend, 2010; Dorsey et al., 2019). When looking at work through an occupational lens, the *OTPF-4* (AOTA, 2020) expands on the notion of work as an occupation to include creating and producing things while maintaining required work-related skills and performance patterns; managing interpersonal relationships; initiating, sustaining, and completing work in a timely manner; complying with work norms and procedures; seeking and responding to feedback and performance; and advocating for oneself in the workplace. Furthermore, there is a temporal component to performance patterns associated with work occupations that may be viewed as organizing, such as in the case of an adolescent who routinely completes their homework immediately after school (AOTA, 2020; Eklund et al., 2017; Larson & Zemke, 2003). It is for these reasons that the work of a student includes academics, volunteerism, and preparation for vocational training.

COMMON CORE AND
STATE EDUCATIONAL STANDARDS

In the late 1970s and early 1980s and in alignment with the social calls for educational opportunity for children with disabilities that led to the passage of the U.S. landmark 1975 Education for all Handicapped Children Act, now called the *IDEA*, accountability in health care and education was becoming paramount. The Agency for Healthcare Research and Quality (2022) established standards that required health care organizations to produce evidence to make health care safer, more accessible, equitable, and affordable and improve outcomes for health care consumers. The U.S. Department of Health and Human Services (2022) called for the development of quality measures across the disciplines to advance the depth, breadth, and translation of knowledge; close the gap in the use of scientific information; and measure and advocate for outcomes and value. The U.S. DOE published *A Nation at Risk: National Commission on Excellence in Education*, which was considered by many to be a rallying cry for educational reform (Bill of Rights Institute, 2022). The report suggested that the U.S. workforce was failing to compete in the global economy and the educational system lacked an effective and universal strategy to meet the needs of the system's stakeholders. To advance educational practices and improve educational outcomes, the U.S. DOE followed the pathways set by the health care industry and began to establish quality indicators and minimum standards of education.

By the late 1980s, the U.S. DOE adopted an array of policies that guided the development of accountability practices for federal and state educational agencies. The Educational Assessment Center and the National Center for Educational Statistics developed educational achievement indicators, and the National Science Foundation commissioned research in indicators of quality education in science and math. These best practice models informed policy and practice decisions and led to the development of common educational standards (Common Core State Standards Initiative, 2022).

In response to this call, all states have adopted educational standards that guide educational programming for students enrolled in public education within the state. Forty-one states across the United States have adopted Common Core State Standards, which prescribe academic standards in math and English language arts/literacy by grade (Common Core State Standards Initiative, 2022). The Common Core State Standards were developed for the purpose of ensuring that students within the United States and its territories graduate from high school with the skills and knowledge necessary to achieve success in postsecondary education, vocational pursuits, careers, and the community (Collette et al., 2017; Common Core State Standards Initiative, 2022). In classrooms around the country, a general education model is used to support all students in meeting the Common Core State Standards. Common Core State Standards can be found on the U.S. or state DOE website.

MULTITIERED SYSTEM OF SUPPORTS

The Multitiered System of Supports (MTSS) is a public health, data-driven, framework that fosters interdisciplinary problem solving to improve outcomes for all students. It uses evidence-based interventions provided on a continuum across three tiers and is matched to the students' needs (Center on Positive Behavioral Interventions and Supports, n.d.). The MTSS follows the principles of Universal Design for Learning (UDL). UDL is a research-based framework that provides educational practice guidance to meet the needs of all students. It provides flexibility and reduces barriers for students. Educational material may be presented in diverse ways, aiding students in demonstrating their knowledge and skills in a variety of ways, and it reduces barriers using educational accommodations without compromising high standards for students (CAST, Inc., 2021; Higher Education Opportunity Act, 2008; Marlin et al., 2022; McMahon & Walker, 2019). UDL supports inclusive educational material creation and the application of it in an educational context (AOTA, 2017a; CAST, Inc., 2021). UDL fosters participation and inclusion in educational occupations (AOTA, 2017a; CAST, Inc., 2021; Higher Education Opportunity Act, 2008). Occupational therapy practitioners can play a key role in supporting the implementation of UDL and MTSS principles in the educational setting by using their knowledge base, activity analysis, and adaptation skills to recommend, educate/train, and apply technology and other methods to foster learning, performance, and participation in the context of the school environment (AOTA, 2017a).

The use of a public health approach to engage in school-wide programming allows occupational therapists to reach more students earlier and prevent some of them from requiring more intensive services later (AOTA et al., 2014; Bazyk & Cahill, 2014; Grajo et al., 2018; Handley-More et al., 2019; Seruya & Garfinkel, 2018); however, only 40% of school-based therapists reported that they engage in MTSS programming (Seruya & Garfinkel, 2020). Within school contexts, occupational therapists support the establishment or restoration of the student's ability to perform school-related activities; modify the environment, adapt tasks, and/or teach compensatory strategies; facilitate habits and routines to support the student–worker role within the domain of occupation; promote the use of assistive technologies that support the student's access to and participation in their schoolwork-related tasks; collaborate with stakeholders to educate and advocate on the student's behalf; and support a student's transition from school to work outside of the school environment, also known as *postsecondary transition* (AOTA, 2017b; Grajo et al., 2020).

SPECIAL EDUCATION SERVICES ALIGNMENT

As described in Chapter 2, educational regulation responded to political and social activism (civil rights), parental and constituency advocacy, congressional findings, and litigious pressures, and over the years of review, amendment, and reauthorization, an array of accountability measures were adopted that align and ensure the following (IDEA, 2004; Every Student Succeeds Act, 2015):

- Children with disabilities are educated in their neighborhood schools in regular classrooms with their nondisabled peers to the greatest extent possible.
- Interdisciplinary teams of educational professionals, specialists, and caregivers work together to evaluate educational access and learning, plan intervention, and collaboratively implement instruction using the best available evidence.
- Progress is monitored, outcomes are measured, and data are used to drive educational decision making.
- Educational achievement, high school graduation, and employment rates rise among individuals with disabilities.

With the guidance of the *OTPF-4* and occupational therapy's theoretical foundations, occupational therapy practitioners are well equipped to address the educational needs of students and those who instruct them in educational settings (AOTA, 2020; World Federation of Occupational Therapists, 2012). Using the full scope of occupational therapy practice, occupational therapy practitioners meet the occupational needs of children and youth across the life span from early childhood through transition to postsecondary environments. We identify and prioritize the occupational strengths, interests, and needs of students using ecological evaluation practices and formal and standardized assessments that target meaningful occupational engagement and participation. We provide services to students in naturally occurring locations and during naturally occurring activities and design intervention using the best available evidence to address the gap between performance and contextual supports by engaging student strengths and modifying environments and tasks. Occupational therapy practitioners collect and analyze data to inform decision making and measure and report outcomes. Handley-More and colleagues (2013) described contextually based and collaborative measures as being two key best practices that align occupational therapy practice and current educational regulation, policy, and guidance.

Contextual Services

Contextual services are services that are provided to students during naturally occurring activities in their naturally occurring environments (Handley-More et al., 2013; Seruya & Garfinkel, 2018). Contextual services are provided across school environments and settings to include classrooms, cafeteria, music room, art room, physical education gym, computer classroom, and the playground. Although providing services in the least restrictive environment is required by IDEA, it is also grounded in an occupation-based practice and supported by the *OTPF-4* (AOTA, 2020; Seruya & Garfinkel, 2018). Many positive outcomes have been noted in the provision of contextual services to include the following (Handley-More et al., 2013):

- Occupational therapy practitioners have the opportunity to model interventions, accommodations, and modifications for instructional staff.
- Interventions are more likely to be carried over by instructional staff and caregivers.
- Learned skills are used more frequently and in more generalized settings.
- Specialized therapy equipment is less likely to be needed because typical classroom materials are used instead.

Collaborative Services

Hanft and Swinth (2011) defined collaborative service as "an interactive process that focuses teams and agencies on enhancing the functional performance, education achievement, and participation of infants/toddlers, children and youth with disabilities" (p. 2). Once again mandated by IDEA for Individualized Education Program (IEP) teams, collaborative services are also supported in occupational guidance and in the *OTPF-4* (AOTA, 2020). Teachers, family members, occupational therapy practitioners, and all other relevant staff collaborate with the students through the referral, evaluation, eligibility determination, goal setting, instruction/intervention, and outcome measurement process to support student access, participation, and benefit from the educational program. Notable outcomes of collaborative services are as follows (Friedman et al., 2023; Handley-More et al., 2013; Sayers, 2008):

- Shared decision making and responsibility for measuring progress and achieving student outcomes
- Shared expertise, skills, and resources across the team
- Greater teacher satisfaction with services and improved carryover of suggestions
- Teachers, parents, administrators, and other stakeholders have an improved understanding of the role and contributions of occupational therapy

SCHOOLWORK OCCUPATIONS

Children in kindergarten through 12th grade are typically expected to engage in schoolwork occupations that involve traditional literacy (reading and writing), math, social studies, science, and technology (Grajo et al., 2020). Schoolwork also includes the ability to demonstrate knowledge in specific subject areas through written, oral, and/or other mediums. Children and adolescents in public schools are generally expected to demonstrate their knowledge by taking tests/examinations using a pencil/pen and paper and/or through the use of a computer or laptop as well (Grajo et al., 2020). Impairments in the traditional literacy skills of reading and writing have been associated with decreased performance and participation in other academic and work-related areas (Grajo et al., 2020; Santangel & Graham, 2016). Table 9-1 illustrates the typical schoolwork tasks, school motor tasks, and school social participation tasks required of students across the educational trajectory.

EDUCATIONAL TRANSITIONS

Occupational therapists are distinctly prepared to be valuable members of a postsecondary transition team. They support students who are transitioning from high school to acquire the skills needed for employment, higher education, and/or independent living (AOTA, 2017b, 2018; Dell'Armo & Tassé, 2019; Majeski et al., 2019). Research shows that by including vocational (work) and functional skills training to students in high school, it prepares them for productive employment in the future (Dell'Armo & Tassé, 2019; Pierce et al., 2020; Wong et al., 2021). Transition services are mandated by IDEA for youth 14 to 21 years of age (IDEA, 2004). Incorporating vocational experiences in school-based practice with a younger population could encourage occupational therapy practitioners to integrate more work-related, occupation-focused interventions to help students achieve their IEP goals (DiMeo, 2022; Giordanella et al., 2015).

TABLE 9-1

Typical Schoolwork Tasks, School Motor Tasks, and School Social Participation Tasks

	SCHOOLWORK TASKS	SCHOOL MOTOR TASKS	SCHOOL PARTICIPATION TASKS
EARLY CHILDHOOD/ PRESCHOOL	Attention regulation in groups Exploration of environment Management of routines	Activity modulation Self-maintenance—basic self-care routines	Cooperative play Sharing and conflict resolution
EARLY ELEMENTARY	Visual discrimination and visual motor integration Trial and error learning Task planning and self-monitoring Overriding sensory data	Eye-hand coordination, stabilization, and praxis Gross motor efficacy	Making "special" friends Developing reciprocity in relationships
LATE ELEMENTARY	Motor persistence and task completion Spatial and sequential planning Experiential learning	Motor memory and visual motor accuracy Planning simple motor sequences First comparisons of athletic capacity	Developing appreciation for the perspectives of others Expanding verbal pragmatics
MIDDLE SCHOOL	Extended mental and motor effort and rapid motor responsivity Material management and organization Critical thinking with manual problem-solving (procedural) learning	Convergence of body image and motor capacities Graphomotor fluency and automaticity Gross motor anticipatory planning	Increasing complexity of thought and expression Compare and contrast ideas
HIGH SCHOOL	Production meta-analysis (previewing, pacing, and self-monitoring) Process-oriented reasoning/production Synthesis of knowledge from experience	Graphomotor fluency and automaticity Gross motor specialization	Intimacy vs. isolation

CASE STUDY

To illustrate the occupations of education and work in a school setting, we explore the case of Laura, a 15-year-old adolescent girl attending a public high school. Laura is diagnosed with a learning disability that affects her ability to read and write with fluency. Throughout elementary and middle school, Laura struggled with academic work involving the written word. She, like all the other children in her kindergarten class, benefited from tablets and headphones that allowed Laura to read books. She and her classmates were provided with a variety of writing tools, such as mini whiteboards, markers, pencils of different shapes and sizes, and pencil grips. When Laura's reading and writing challenges interfered more with her ability to get her work done, the MTSS team, which included an occupational therapist, met at regular intervals to discuss Laura's strengths and challenges as determined by standardized general education assessments. Some of the strategies were increased use of a tablet and headphones during reading lessons, having an alphabet card taped inside her notebook for easy reference, small-group instruction, and, eventually, more individualized literacy instruction by the general education teacher. By the end of first grade, Laura was referred to special education, and an IEP was developed for her based on her needs at the time. She has continued to receive special education services for reading and math through her elementary, middle, and high school years. Table 9-2 provides details on Laura's occupational profile.

Organizing Model of Practice: Person-Environment-Occupation Model

The organizing model of practice used in Laura's case is the Person-Environment-Occupation (PEO) model (Law et al.,1996), which was described in detail in Chapter 6. By focusing on the relationship between Laura, her school-related environments, and her occupations, the occupational therapist can choose from a broad range of assessments and interventions targeting one or more of the three components of the model. Laura's personal skills may be evaluated using a variety of skill-based assessments, such as evaluations that target visual perceptual skills or motor functioning; however, they do not give an accurate picture of Laura's overall functioning. An occupation-based approach to assessment is supported through the PEO model as well. When assessing function and Laura's ability to perform work-based occupations, an occupation-based assessment captures Laura's functioning within the context of the environment in which she is performing actual occupations. Occupation-based evaluations may not be able to identify the root cause of an individual's functional challenges; however, it gives a more holistic view of occupational challenges. Interventions provided when using the PEO model target occupations rather than individual personal skill development. Best practice within the school environment includes interventions that target occupations in natural environments by providing a "just right challenge" for the student and considers the student's strengths, challenges, beliefs, and motivators (AOTA, 2017a, 2020; Bazyk & Cahill, 2014; Cahill & Beisbier, 2020; Seruya & Garfinkel, 2020).

The reason that the PEO model was chosen for Laura is that it differs from other ecological models in that it accounts for changing circumstances or situations and proposes that because there is a dynamic component to this model, there is a need for ongoing monitoring of interventions because one or more of the three components of the model (i.e., person, environment, or occupation) may change (Law et al., 1996). Laura is an adolescent, and her personal skills will continue to change as she continues to mature and her needs change. Environmental modifications will change based on where she is performing her educational and academic tasks, transitional support activities, work, and the nature of the schoolwork in which she is engaging.

TABLE 9-2

Laura's Occupational Profile

What concerns do Laura and her team have about her occupational engagement?	As a 15-year-old high school student, Laura is continuing to receive special education services targeting her literacy-based learning disability. She is struggling to complete her academic work as the complexity of the curriculum increases. The team has expressed concerns in her ability to complete academic work and is concerned for her postsecondary transition.
In what occupations is Laura successful, and what barriers impact her success?	Laura is highly engaging with adults and peers alike and is motivated to engage in the occupations that her peers are typically involved in. She manages her self-care needs independently, and she can access public transportation with the assistance of her peers. She struggles with tasks involving reading and math skills. Academic learning is an educational occupation that Laura struggles with because of her challenges in the areas of reading and writing. Laura is facing barriers to accessing printed materials; she struggles to take notes and to express herself in a written fashion.
What is Laura's occupational history?	Laura has been receiving special education support for her learning challenges in reading and math since the first grade. She enjoys interacting with her peers (both face-to-face and on her phone) and playing sports. Schoolwork tasks are not favored, but she will engage in them as necessary. She enjoys taking care of herself (trying out new hairstyles) and her beloved dog, Buddy.
What are Laura's and her team's personal interests and values?	Laura and her team want to continue to support her academic achievement and her transition to postsecondary education. Laura wants to engage in a volunteer activity, which is required of her school and a top interest of her peers.

(continued)

TABLE 9-2 (CONTINUED)
Laura's Occupational Profile

What aspects of the contexts do Laura and her team see as supporting engagement in desired occupations, and what aspects are inhibiting engagement?	
ENVIRONMENT	Laura has a supportive peer group and strong family support. Volunteerism is a work-related occupation that all students in Laura's school are required to engage in before graduation. She decided to volunteer at a soup kitchen across town; however, the only way for her to travel there is by bus. Taking a bus to the soup kitchen with a classmate is an option, but the classmate no longer goes to the soup kitchen the same days as Laura, and Laura is unable to read the bus schedule independently.
PERSONAL	Laura has expressed an interest in working in her family's restaurant after high school. She and her transition planning team, which includes an occupational therapist, have begun preparing for Laura's transition for 1 year. In the state where Laura resides, postsecondary transition planning begins at age 14 years and continues through graduation or age 21 years. Postsecondary transition planning is documented on Laura's IEP.
PERFORMANCE PATTERNS	Laura is experiencing greater challenges related to her learning disability. She is finding it harder to be successful because the demands of her education and work occupations have increased; therefore, Laura has been referred to the school district's occupational therapist for support.

(continued)

TABLE 9-2 (CONTINUED)
Laura's Occupational Profile

What client factors do Laura and her team see as supporting engagement in desired occupations, and what aspects are inhibiting engagement?	
VALUES, BELIEFS, AND SPIRITUALITY	Laura has supportive family members who have been strong advocates for her throughout her school years. She is actively involved in her social group and the community and looking forward to a volunteer experience. Laura has difficulty completing tasks involving reading and math.
BODY FUNCTIONS	Laura is involved actively in occupations that promote physical activity. She has difficulty with reading and math.
BODY STRUCTURES	Laura is motivated to use compensatory strategies to support her literacy functioning. Many of her peers use applications (apps) to support independence in literacy and community mobility. Laura will need support in the use of compensatory strategies to support her academic achievement and to support volunteerism and postsecondary transition.
What are Laura's and her team's priorities and desired goals?	
OCCUPATIONAL PERFORMANCE	Laura has a strong desire to participate in the occupations that her peers engage in. She is motivated to learn and has begun expressing ideas for her future.
PREVENTION	Laura's team would like to see her independently use compensatory strategies to promote safe and independent learning, transition to work, and community mobility.
HEALTH AND WELLNESS	Laura engages in a healthy and active lifestyle and wants to establish the tools to continue to engage in her physical and social environment independently.
QUALITY OF LIFE AND WELL-BEING	Laura, her family, and her school team want to continue her progression toward academic and volunteerism independence to increase her outlooks for postsecondary education and employment success.
PARTICIPATION AND ROLE COMPETENCE	Laura is motivated to learn and engage in activities required of her schoolwork and postsecondary transition.
OCCUPATIONAL JUSTICE	Laura, her family, and her school team want to ensure that she has the skills to be a successful and productive participant in her community.

Adapted from American Occupational Therapy Association. (2020). AOTA occupational profile template. https://www.aota.org/-/media/Corporate/Files/Practice/Manage/Documentation/AOTA-Occupational-Profile-Template.pdf

Strengths and Challenges

One of the core values of the field of occupational therapy is that our assessments and interventions be occupation based (AOTA, 2020). Using the PEO model, we assess the personal factors that may impact the student's ability to complete their occupations. We investigate the characteristics of the environment/context within which the student will be performing their academic and work-based occupations, and we analyze the occupation and activities that the student must perform as part of their school-based work (Law et al., 1996). Collaboration with school-based stakeholders is critical to serving children and youth in their natural environments and contexts, providing training with feedback and follow-up, and supporting the best student outcomes (Cahill & Beisbier, 2020; Seruya & Garfinkel, 2020).

Early in Laura's school career, her occupational therapist(s) administered assessments designed to capture Laura's strengths and challenges. They used the School Function Assessment (Coster et al., 1998), which is a criterion-referenced, multidisciplinary, occupation-based evaluation tool. When completing the School Function Assessment, the school-based team, which may consist of the teacher and related service providers, collaborates to complete the assessment and to gather information about the student's specific performance and engagement in school-based occupations (Coster et al., 1998). It is necessary at times, as was the case with Laura, to delve deeper into specific skill areas to determine a student's baseline of function. Laura was given a visual perceptual assessment for the purpose of gaining more information about Laura's visual perceptual skills because they are an especially crucial factor in literacy and reading. Through the collaboration with the team, the school nurse indicated that Laura's vision and hearing are intact. Therefore, those two performance skill areas could be ruled out as the root cause for Laura's difficulty with reading and writing.

Complementary Models of Practice

Although the PEO model provided the basic framework for Laura's assessment and intervention, two complementary models of practice are also used in the case of Laura: the Model of Human Occupation (MOHO) and the Four-Quadrant Model of Facilitated Learning (4QM). In addition, the Student-Environment-Task-Technology (SETT) framework is used to introduce and promote the use of assistive technology in her school day. These models enhance the effectiveness of Laura's outcomes.

Model of Human Occupation

MOHO expands on the PEO model in that it considers how occupations are motivated, patterned, and performed within everyday contexts (Kielhofner, 2008). The MOHO model provides a means to describe how people develop and modify their occupations as they interact with the environment. This dynamic systems model uses information from the environment, considered input. This information is then processed through three subsystems: volition, habituation, and performance. The volition subsystem describes how the individual initiates action, and it includes personal causation, or a person's sense of effectiveness and confidence when participating in an action. Interests are an individual's desire and intention to seek pleasurable emotions from specific actions, objects, or events. Valued goals are how an individual determines the importance of different occupational behaviors; they are the outcome. The habituation subsystem is responsible for daily routines and patterns of behavior as well as the sequence of performing actions. After the interaction between the input and the three subsystems, the dynamic system generates output in the form of information and action. This output provides feedback to the dynamic system and becomes new input through a feedback loop (Kielhofner, 2008).

Laura's motivation to use compensatory strategies is key to her success in her educational and work-related occupations. Small-group service delivery methods that were used throughout Laura's school career provide an opportunity for increased motivation and modeling (Cahill & Beisbier, 2020). An occupation-based assessment tool that aligns with MOHO is the Canadian Occupational Performance Measure (Law et al., 2014). The Canadian Occupational Performance Measure is a client-centered and evidence-based outcome measure that explores self-perception of an individual regarding their participation and performance in daily life over time (Law et al., 2014).

Four-Quadrant Model of Facilitated Learning

The 4QM informs an occupational therapist's clinical reasoning when using teaching-learning approaches (Greber et al., 2007). Like the PEO model, it is based on the changing needs of the learner during the acquisition of new skills. The first quadrant in the 4QM is direct, explicit instruction by the occupational therapist. The second quadrant involves the therapist providing hints or cues, even questions, to prompt the student in the learning process. The third quadrant shifts the focus of the learning to the student. The student uses strategies such as the use of mnemonics or the use of verbal self-talk to facilitate the learning process. The fourth quadrant in the 4QM involves the student reflecting on their own performance, and it may include the ability to self-correct.

The 4QM can be used to frame Laura's learning experiences based on her dynamic learning needs. For example, when beginning to learn an innovative technology, such as the use of built-in accessibility features on a smartphone, the occupational therapist provides direct instruction to Laura (first quadrant). After three sessions, the therapist provides hints and cues to help Laura to remember the sequence of turning on the "read aloud" feature on her phone (second quadrant). After five sessions, Laura begins using self-talk to remember the sequence of turning on the built-in feature (third quadrant). During the eighth session, Laura reflects meaningfully on her ability to use the technology effectively (fourth quadrant).

Student-Environment-Task-Technology Framework

Moving forward, in the case of Laura, it may be necessary for her to use assistive technology to facilitate success in her work-related occupations. Elements of the PEO model, which are at the very core of the profession of occupational therapy (AOTA, 2020), align with complementary models targeting assistive technology–based decision making. A decision-making model that is specifically focused on students is the SETT framework (Zabala, 2005).

When using the SETT framework (Zabala, 2005), S refers to student factors, strengths, and challenges; E refers to the environment or context within which the student will be expected to perform their occupation; the first T refers to the characteristics of the task or occupation; and the final T refers to the characteristics of the technology to be used. Zabala (2005) developed this model for assessment to indicate the importance of matching the student, environment/context, and task/occupation to the technology. The SETT assistive technology decision-making model shares common constructs of the person, environment, activity or task, and technology, and provides a framework to support practitioners in the assistive technology decision-making process, which aligns with the OTPF-4 (AOTA et al., 2014; AOTA, 2016). It is important to note that the success of the assistive technology intervention lies in the occupational therapist's ability to analyze, problem solve, and understand the dynamic person-occupation-intervention relationship, not simply the characteristics of the piece of assistive technology itself (AOTA, 2016).

Because Laura is having difficulty reading bus maps/schedules when going to her volunteer placement, the occupational therapist and the vocational counselor collaborated to determine if assistive technology would support her participation in her volunteer work. They used the SETT framework to determine if there was a need for assistive technology and, if so, what type of technology would best fit her needs. To gather information pertinent to the student (S) areas of the SETT framework, Laura's occupational therapist completed a comprehensive occupational therapy evaluation, identifying Laura's areas of strength and her areas of challenge. Also identified during the evaluation was Laura's desire to not appear different from her peers and the fact that she and her family have limited financial resources. The occupational therapist observed the environments (E) and contexts in which Laura would need to potentially use a piece of assistive technology to help her read a bus schedule. The task (T) identified as being challenging was reading a bus schedule. The occupational therapist identified both high- and low-tech tools (T) that could potentially support Laura's participation by overcoming the barrier of reading a bus map to get to her volunteer position. As they collaborated, it was determined that given Laura's skill set and the tools and resources that she has available, using her smartphone would work best for her. Laura's desire to not appear different from her peers was taken into consideration in the decision-making process. The assistive technology chosen uses everyday technologies that are available to all students, thereby assuring that while using the accessibility features on her phone, Laura would not appear different from her peers. In fact, many of Laura's friends use these features on their devices as well, making Laura feel more included in her peer interactions, which reinforces her motivation to use the assistive technology (Kielhofner, 2008). IDEA (2004) and the Assistive Technology Act of 2004 are two pieces of legislation that promote access to assistive technology for individuals with disabilities to participate in education, employment, and everyday activities more fully. The use of these specific tools is listed on Laura's IEP as necessary assistive technology. The potential goal areas developed by Laura and her occupational therapist are as follows:

- Laura will participate in sessions with the occupational therapist in the vocational counseling center to foster collaboration with the vocational rehabilitation counselor who is supporting Laura during her volunteer placement.
- Intervention techniques to achieve the goal of using the built-in read aloud feature on her phone will be occupation based. Laura will practice using the technology for its intended purpose.
- Laura will download the transit app during an occupational therapy session. She will navigate the different sections on the app and locate the schedule section. She will practice finding schedules that match the days and times when she will be volunteering.
- Laura's parents and her vocational rehabilitation counselor will be educated and trained in the use of the technology used by Laura to support carryover.

Once Laura achieves mastery of the use of the technology, the occupational therapist will periodically reassess her needs for assistive technology.

CONCLUSION

Although the primary occupation of students in school is education (AOTA, 2020; Frolek Clark & Ponsolle-Mays, 2019) wherein students engage in academic and nonacademic pursuits, extracurricular, and technologic activities (AOTA, 2020), work is another important school-based occupation for young students and adolescents. Used in this context, work includes creating and producing things, such as curriculum-based projects; managing interpersonal relationships within the social context of school; initiating, sustaining, and completing work in a timely manner; and advocating for oneself within the educational realm (AOTA, 2020). To illustrate how the occupations of education and work relate to students in school, the case of Laura, a 15-year-old with learning disabilities, was presented along with organizing models of practice to demonstrate how interventions in these two school-based occupations are rooted in theory.

REFERENCES

Agency for Healthcare Research and Quality. (2022). About AHRQ. https://www.ahrq.gov/cpi/about/index.html

American Occupational Therapy Association. (2016). Assistive technology and occupational performance. *American Journal of Occupational Therapy, 70,* 7012410030. http://doi.org/10.5014/ajot.2016.706S02

American Occupational Therapy Association. (2017a). Guidelines for occupational therapy services in early intervention and schools. *American Journal of Occupational Therapy, 71*(Suppl. 2), 7112410010. https://doi.org/10.5014/ajot.2017.716S01

American Occupational Therapy Association. (2017b). Occupational therapy services in facilitating work participation and performance. *American Journal of Occupational Therapy, 71*(Suppl. 2), 7112410040. https://doi.org/10.5014/ajot.716S05

American Occupational Therapy Association. (2018). *Transitions for children and youth: How occupational therapy can help.* https://www.aota.org/-/media/Corporate/Files/AboutOT/Professionals/WhatIsOT/CY/Fact-Sheets/Transitions.pdf

American Occupational Therapy Association. (2020). Occupational therapy practice framework: Domain and process (4th ed.). *American Journal of Occupational Therapy, 74*(Suppl. 2), 7412410010p1-7412410010p87. https://doi.org/10.5014/ajot.2020.74S2001

American Occupational Therapy Association, American Physical Therapy Association, & American Speech-Language-Hearing Association. (2014). *Workload approach: A paradigm shift for positive impact on student outcomes.* https://www.asha.org/siteassets/practice-portal/caseloadworkload/apta-asha-aota-joint-doc-workload-approach-schools.pdf

Assistive Technology Act of 2004, Pub. L. 108-364, 118 Stat. 1707 (2004).

Bazyk, S., & Cahill, S. (2014). School-based occupational therapy. In J. Case-Smith & J. C. O'Brien (Eds.), *Occupational therapy for children and adolescents* (7th ed., pp. 665-703). Elsevier Mosby.

Bill of Rights Institute. (2022). A nation at risk: Responsibility and the National Commission on Excellence in Education – handout A: Narrative. https://billofrightsinstitute.org/activities/a-nation-at-risk-responsibility-and-the-national-commission-on-excellence-in-education-handout-a-narrative

Cahill, S. M., & Beisbier, S. (2020). Occupational therapy practice guidelines for children and youth ages 5-21 years. *American Journal of Occupational Therapy, 74*(4), 7404397010p1-7404397010p48. https://doi.org/10.5014/ajot.2020.744001

CAST, Inc. (2021). The UDL guidelines. https://udlguidelines.cast.org/?utm_source=castsite&lutm_medium=web&utm_campaign=none&utm_content=aboutudl

Center on Positive Behavioral Interventions and Supports. (n.d.). Tiered PBIS framework. https://www.pbis.org/pbis/tiered-framework

Christiansen, C. H., & Townsend, E. A. (2010). *Introduction to occupation: The art and science of living* (2nd ed.). Pearson Education.

Collette, D., Anson, K., Halabi, N., Schlierman, A., & Suriner, A. (2017). Handwriting and Common Core State Standards: Teacher, occupational therapist, and administrator perceptions from New York State public schools. *American Journal of Occupational Therapy, 71,* 7106220010. https://doi.org/10.5014/ajot.2017.021808

Common Core State Standards Initiative. (2022). About the standards. https://www.thecorestandards.org/about-the-standards/

Coster, W. J., Deeney, T. A., Haltiwanger, J. T., & Haley, S. M. (1998). *School function assessment.* Psychological Corporation/Therapy Skill Builders.

Dell'Armo, K. A., & Tassé, M. J. (2019). The role of adaptive behavior and parent expectations in predicting post-school outcomes for young adults with intellectual disability. *Journal of Autism & Developmental Disorders, 49,* 1638-1651. https://doi.org/10.1007/s10803-018-3857-6

DiMeo, S. (2022). Implementing the early skills vocational program in school-based occupational therapy practice. *SIS Quarterly Practice Connections, 7*(2), 2-4.

Dorsey, J., Ehrenfried, H., Finch, D., & Jaegers, L. (2019). *Work.* In B. A. B. Schell & G. Gillen (Eds.), *Willard and Spackman's occupational therapy* (13th ed., pp. 779-804). Wolters Kluwer.

Eklund, M., Orban, K., Argentzell, E., Bejerholm, U., Tjörnstrand, C., Erlandsson, L. K., & Hakansson, C. (2017). The linkage between patterns of daily occupations and occupational balance: Applications within occupational science and occupational therapy practice. *Scandinavian Journal of Occupational Therapy, 24*, 41-56. https://doi.org/10.1080/11038128.2016.1224271

Every Student Succeeds Act, 20 U.S.C. § 6301 (2015). https://www.congress.gov/bill/114th-congress/senate-bill/1177

Friedman, Z. L., Hubbard, H., & Seruya, F. M. (2023). Building better teams: Impact of education and coaching intervention on interprofessional collaboration between teachers and occupational therapists in schools. *Journal of Occupational Therapy, Schools, & Early Intervention, 16*(2), 173-193. https://doi.org/10.1080/19411243.2022.2037492

Frolek Clark, G., & Ponsolle-Mays, M. (2019). The OTPF-3: Communicating occupational therapy in schools. In G. F. Clark, J. E. Fioux, B. E. Chandler, & J. Cashman (Eds.), *Best practices for occupational therapy in schools* (2nd ed.). AOTA Press/The American Occupational Therapy Association, Inc.

Giordanella, D., Dulanie, J., Chubet, C., Rotko, C., & Seruya, F. M. (2015). Practitioners' perceptions of occupational therapy in middle school settings. *American Journal of Occupational Therapy, 69*(Suppl. 1), 6911510129. https://doi.org/10.5014/ajot.2015.69S1-RP203B

Grajo, L. C., Candler, C., & Sarafian, A. (2020). Interventions within the scope of occupational therapy to improve children's academic participation: A systematic review. *American Journal of Occupational Therapy, 74*(2), 7402180030p1-7402180030p32. https://doi.org/10.5014/ajot.2020.039016

Grajo, L., Schefkind, S., Collette, D., Frauwirth, S., Garfinkel, M., Handley-More, D., Hardman, L., Hinerfeld, D., & Lucas, C. (2018, April). *Beyond handwriting: Advocating for the role of occupational therapy in supporting literacy.* Workshop presented at the AOTA Annual Conference & Expo, Salt Lake City, UT.

Greber, C., Ziviani, J., & Rodger, S. (2007). The Four-Quadrant Model of facilitated learning (part 1): Using teaching–learning approaches in occupational therapy. *Australian Occupational Therapy Journal, 54*(Suppl. 1), S31-S39.

Handley-More, D., Bruegger, T., Costello, P., & Garfinkel, M. (2019, April). *Exploring the role of occupational therapy in supporting literacy across the lifespan.* Paper presented at the AOTA Annual Conference & Expo, New Orleans, LA.

Handley-More, D., Wall, E., Orentlicher, M. L., & Hollenbeck, J. (2013). Working in early intervention and school settings: Current views of best practice. *Early Intervention & School Special Interest Section Quarterly, 20*(2), 1-4.

Hanft, B., & Swinth, Y. (2011). Editorial: Community on collaboration. *Journal of Occupational Therapy, Schools, & Early Intervention, 4*, 2-7.

Higher Education Opportunity Act, 20 U.S.C. § 1001 et seq. (2008). https://www2.ed.gov/policy/highered/leg/hea08/index.html

Individuals with Disabilities Education Act of 2004, Pub. L. 108-446, 20 U.S.C. § 1400 et seq (2004).

Kielhofner, G. (2008). *The Model of Human Occupation: Theory and application* (4th ed.). Lippincott Williams & Wilkins.

Larson, E. A., & Zemke, R. (2003). Shaping the temporal patterns of our lives: The social coordination of occupation. *Journal of Occupational Science, 10*, 80-89. https://doi.org/10.1080/14427591.2003.9686514

Law, M., Baptiste, S., Carswell, A., McColl, M. A., Polatajko, H., & Pollock, N. (2014). *Canadian Occupational Performance Measure* (5th ed.). CAOT Publications.

Law, M., Cooper, B., Strong, S., Stewart, D., Rigby, P., & Letts, L. (1996). The Person-Environment-Occupation Model: A transactive approach to occupational performance. *Canadian Journal of Occupational Therapy, 63*, 9-23. http://doi.org/10.1177/000841749606300103

Majeski, K., Hollebeck, J., Berg, L. A., Spence, A., Mankey, T. A., Carroll, T., & Rudd, L. (2019). Supporting secondary transition planning through evaluation: Occupational therapy's distinct value. *OT Practice, 24*(1), 19-25.

Marlin, A. L., Fletcher, T. S., & Garcia, N. M. (2022). A recipe for session success: Promoting OT through Universal Design for Learning and text analysis. https://www.aota.org/publications/ot-practice/ot-practice-issues/2022/universal-design-learning-text-analysis/open-universal-design-learning-text-analysis

McMahon, D., & Walker, Z. (2019). Leveraging emerging technology to design an inclusive future with universal design for learning. *Career Development and Transition for Exceptional Individuals, 42*(2), 99-110. https://doi.org/10.26529/cepsj.639

Pierce, D., Sakemiller, L., Spence, A., & LoBianco, T. (2020). Effectiveness of transition readiness interventions by school-based occupational therapy personnel. *OTJR: Occupation, Participation & Health, 40*(1), 27-35. https://doi.org/10.1177/1539449219850129

Santangel, T., & Graham, S. (2016). A comprehensive meta-analysis of handwriting instruction. *Educational Psychology Review, 28*, 225-265. https://doi.org/10.1007/s10648-015-9335-1

Sayers, B. R. (2008). Collaboration in school settings: A critical appraisal of the topic. *Journal of Occupational Therapy, Schools, & Early Intervention, 1*, 170-179.

Seruya, F. M., & Garfinkel, M. (2018). Implementing contextually based services: Where do we begin? *SIS Quarterly Practice Connections, 3*(3), 4-7.

Seruya, F. M., & Garfinkel, M. (2020). Caseload and workload: Current trends in school-based practice across the United States. *American Journal of Occupational Therapy, 74*, 7405205090. https://doi.org/10.5014/ajot.2020.039818

U.S. Department of Health and Human Services. (2022). Quality measures development overview. https://www.hhs.gov/guidance/document/quality-measures-development-overview

Wong, J., Coster, W. J., Cohn, E. S., & Orsmond, G. I. (2021). Identifying school-based factors that predict employment outcomes for transition-age youth with autism spectrum disorder. *Journal of Autism and Developmental Disorders, 51*, 60-74. https://doi.org/10.1007/s10803-020-04515-2

World Federation of Occupational Therapists. (2012). About occupational therapy. https://wfot.org/about/about-occupational-therapy

Zabala, J. S. (2005). Using the SETT framework to level the learning field for students with disabilities. https://ttaconline.org/Resource/JWHaEa5BS762YneJq2Re3Q/Resource-sett-framework-joy-zabala

Play and Leisure

Francine M. Seruya, PhD, OTR/L, FAOTA
and Tina Weisman, OTD, OTR/L

Chapter Objectives

1. Define the occupations of play and leisure as they relate to the context of school-based practice.
2. Identify meaningful engagement in play and leisure as they support students' social and emotional development as well as contribute to their academic experience.
3. Develop a theoretically based evaluation and intervention plan to address engagement in appropriate play and leisure pursuits for school-based settings.

Play and leisure activities are noted to be typical and expected occupations for children and youth (American Occupational Therapy Association [AOTA], 2011). Occupational therapy practitioners frequently use the activity of play as an intervention approach regardless of functional outcome to facilitate active participation when working with children. The ability to engage in play and leisure activities is essential to promote development in a variety of developmental domains (Cahill & Beisbier, 2020).

Laverdure, P., & Seruya, F. M. *Theory in School-Based*
Occupational Therapy Practice: A Practical Application (pp. 135-146).
DOI: 10.4324/9781003526773-10

PLAY

Play has been defined as an activity that is intrinsically motivated, has no defined external rules, contains some element of imagination, and is a relatively stress-free activity in which the participant plays an active role (AOTA, 2020). According to the AOTA, play can be defined as "any spontaneous or organized activity that provides enjoyment, entertainment, amusement or diversion" (Parham & Fazio, 2008, p. 448). In early childhood, infants and toddlers learn about the environment and themselves through their play. As children grow, they begin to participate in more structured types of play such as organized games and sports. They continue to learn about themselves and the world via play activities; however, their play typically begins to increasingly involve individuals outside of their more immediate family circle. As indicated in the fourth edition of *Occupational Therapy Practice Framework: Domain and Process* (*OTPF-4*; AOTA, 2020), play as an occupation can include those activities that involve exploration as well as those that are more participatory in nature. Play exploration includes identification, exploration, practice of play, and engagement in pretend or symbolic play and in games with rules. Participating in play and obtaining, using, and maintaining toys and equipment are indicative of participation (AOTA, 2020).

LEISURE

On the other hand, leisure can refer to any set of activities that are not work or life activities in which people engage in their free time. The AOTA defines leisure as "nonobligatory activity that is intrinsically motivated and engaged in during discretionary time, that is, time not committed to obligatory occupations such as work, self-care, or sleep" (Parham & Fazio, 1997, as cited in AOTA, 2014, p. S21). Therefore, play might be considered a type of leisure activity depending on the context in which it occurs. As children move into adolescence, play can, at times, appear more closely aligned with leisure pursuits, especially when considering the time spent in more free-flowing activities with time just spent together. Like play, the *OTPF-4* recognizes both leisure exploration and leisure participation as components of the occupation, with leisure exploration referring to the exploration and identification of interests, skills, and opportunities for activities and participation including obtaining, maintaining, and using equipment as well as the act of planning and participation in leisure (AOTA, 2020).

PLAY AND LEISURE AS RELATED TO THE SCHOOL SETTING

Although the primary focus in school settings is related to academics, the occupations of play and leisure are integrally woven into the context of the classroom. The use of play is often seen to provide learning activities in a way that is more engaging to children and, therefore, allows them to more actively participate in the learning process. When children initially enter preschool settings, classrooms incorporate a variety of play activities to encourage learning and development via activities such as imaginary play, building activities, and structured games. The use of play and games continues into the primary grades. Children in kindergarten and first grade continue to have imaginary and construction-type activities as part of their daily classroom routines. Frequently, academic concepts are incorporated into play and game-type tasks. For example, when teaching letter identification and formation, the teacher may have children draw letters in shaving cream on a table or glue scraps of paper onto letter templates, or when teaching foundational math skills, the teacher may have children place counting bears into cups.

Children also engage in more structured play in classes such as physical education or when on the playground for recess. Games such as tag, Red Rover, and hide-and-seek all help to teach children about rules as well as turn taking and, depending on the game, may incorporate academic concepts such as counting. As children move into the higher elementary grades, less emphasis is placed on imaginary play, and more structured games and activities are used. For example, a teacher might have timed races to encourage automaticity in basic arithmetic or the use of team games structured around popular games such as Wheel of Fortune or Jeopardy to engage children in mastering content. Children in the higher elementary grades also begin to participate in more organized team sporting activities when in physical education such as games like volleyball, kickball, and softball.

As children move into middle and high school, organized play via team sports continues and oftentimes may also include involvement in teams that are related to but outside of the typical school day. As children move toward their adolescent years, play and leisure are often intertwined via team-building activities in which players are encouraged to participate in activities. Middle school– and high school–age children also begin to engage in more social leisure activities as peer relationships become more valued. Adolescents may begin to engage in activities such as simply spending time together talking, going to events and activities outside the school environment such as to the mall or movies, and other events based on mutual interests. At this age, adolescents become more independent in their play and leisure pursuits and begin to organize and plan events without the assistance of adults.

CASE STUDY

Caroline is a 16-year-old adolescent girl diagnosed with athetoid cerebral palsy. She has fluctuating tone with increased right-sided impairment. She has decreased use of her right arm, which interferes with activities requiring the use of both hands. She lives in an accessible building with her mom and half brother. Caroline has no relationship with her biological father but does occasionally spend time with her stepfather, although he is frequently not home because of his work schedule. She feels very connected to her mother and speaks of her strong religious values as being important in the household. Her home environment includes an accessible apartment, and her mother has a wheelchair-accessible van that has accommodations made specifically for her needs. Caroline's mother worries about her ability to successfully negotiate her chair in the community; therefore, when they go out, her mother manually pushes and directs the chair instead of allowing Caroline to drive it herself.

Academically, Caroline is doing well in school. She is in general education classes with extra support for reading and math. She receives accommodations to have notes provided for her, and she is provided a scribe to complete all written work. Caroline is socially aware and expresses her frustration with her movement impairments impeding her ability to engage in self-care as well as play and leisure pursuits. She reports feelings of low self-esteem and self-worth and states she wants to have more friends. She is an avid football fan and especially wants to be able to go out with friends to see games at her school as well as to hang out with peers to watch games on television.

Caroline has a strong religious background and goes to church weekly with her mother. She believes the church to be important in her life. Caroline's values are highly linked to the teachings of her church, and she feels it is important to be an active member of that community. Caroline identifies going to church weekly and other church events, attending school football games, and socializing with her friends as important extracurricular, leisure activities for her. Although she enjoys these activities, Caroline struggles in relation to her overall level of arousal as well as with emotional regulation when engaged in these less structured environments. She states she often goes through highs and lows, sometimes feeling very energized to engage with friends and at other times struggles to fit in, feeling as though she is much more immature in her behavior. Table 10-1 outlines areas of the occupational profile and Caroline's areas of strength and challenges in each.

Organizing Model of Practice: Occupational Adaptation Model

When reviewing the occupational profile, it is evident that Caroline has definite desires and can articulate the types of goals she has as related to play and leisure pursuits. Her ability to be self-reflective and evaluate her current performance aligns well with the need for assessment of relative mastery noted within the Occupational Adaptation Model (OAM). Further discussion with Caroline also indicates she is aware of the challenges she has engaging in her desired play and leisure occupations, and her innate desire to be able to perform in a more efficient and effective manner also aligns well with the concepts found within the model.

The focus of the OAM is centered on a person's innate drive to participate in occupation and their ability to mitigate, via adaptation, their internal skills and abilities with the environment or context within which the occupation is carried out (Graco, 2017; Schkade & Schultz, 1992). The OAM posits when there is misalignment between the internal, personal factors and the expectations or confines of the context, dysfunction occurs, and there is a breakdown in the ability to participate in meaningful occupations (Schkade & Schultz, 1992). The goal of intervention is to facilitate the child's ability to adapt via changes in strategy or via compensatory approaches to allow for not only participation but also to have engagement in occupation that is personally satisfying (Graco, 2017). The ability to self-reflect and self-evaluate is essential in the OAM to determine if a child has achieved "relative mastery" or a sufficient level of satisfaction with their efficiency and effectiveness in their occupational engagement (Schkade & Schultz, 1992). This feedback is a critical component within the occupational adaptation process. Child-directed goal setting is an essential component of this model because the internal desire to engage is personal and can only be determined by understanding the child's wants and needs in relation to their occupational engagement. The use of occupation as the means of intervention is also crucial because it provides opportunities for active adaptation while engaged in the actual desired occupation (Graco, 2017; Schkade & Schultz, 1992).

Using occupation-based evaluation in conjunction with clinical reasoning based on areas of challenge and strengths, it appears the selection of occupational adaptation as the organizing model of practice is appropriate because it adequately addresses Caroline's ability to engage in occupation, self-reflect, and determine her level of perceived and real satisfaction with her performance as related to her ability to engage in play and leisure-type occupations. Although the organizing model of practice appears to be a good fit for Caroline, there are other challenges she has in relation to client and environmental factors that need further assessment and subsequent interventions that are more targeted. Therefore, the use of other complementary models of practice is warranted.

TABLE 10-1	
Caroline's Occupational Profile	
What concerns do Caroline and her team have about her occupational engagement?	Caroline sets unrealistic long-term transitional goals.
	Caroline exhibits avoidance/defiance behaviors to suggestions that differ from her future predictions.
	Caroline reports that she worries about her mother's well-being and feels like a burden in her life.
	Caroline reports that she is stuck in her home and does not have the support systems to go out in the community like her typical sibling.
	Caroline is resistant to accept help from her care manager.
	Caroline is resistant to solution-based problem solving.
	Caroline is showing signs of depression and helplessness.
In what occupations is Caroline successful, and what barriers impact her success?	Caroline is independent in self-feeding. She requires minimal to moderate assistance to open containers.
	She has limited opportunities to engage in meal preparation at home and within her school setting.
	Caroline navigates her power wheelchair within her school setting with minimal verbal cues negotiating busy hallways. Caroline is independent in operating all display components and features of her power wheelchair. Caroline requires moderate assistance to buckle and unbuckle her seat belt. She requires maximal assistance to move her footplate in preparation for transfers.
	Caroline requires supervision and verbal safety cues for community navigation.
	Caroline has minimal opportunities for community mobility outside of the school campus.
	Caroline is eager to participate in community peer social activities.
	Caroline has limited access to community activities secondary to a lack of transportation, limited caregiver opportunities, and environmental barriers within her community.
What is Caroline's occupational history?	Caroline was born at 32 weeks' gestation and was diagnosed with cerebral palsy at birth. Caroline lives in a small one-bedroom apartment with her mother and half brother. Caroline does not have a relationship with her biological father but spends time with her stepfather. Caroline reports that her mother does not work because "she has to take care of me." Caroline is doing well in her general education classes, requiring additional support for reading and math. Her accommodations include all notes provided for her and a scribe to complete all written work. She is beginning to use talk to text for short homework assignments. She struggles to participate in appropriate play and leisure activities because of motoric and mobility limitations as well as some psychosocial barriers such as emotional lability and difficulty with managing more nuanced social situations.
	(continued)

TABLE 10-1 (CONTINUED)

Caroline's Occupational Profile

What are Caroline's and her team's personal interests and values?	Caroline is active in her church community. She embraces her faith and customs. She enjoys watching football with her mother, brother, and stepfather. She is eager to go to a Giants game with her friends.

What aspects of the contexts do Caroline and her team see as supporting engagement in desired occupations, and what aspects are inhibiting engagement?

	SUPPORTING	INHIBITING
ENVIRONMENT	Accessible apartment and school buildings	Unable to be left unattended because of dependence in self-care, meal preparation, and toileting Requires adult assistance to participate in community activities
PERSONAL	Supportive family, church community, teachers, and related service therapists	Dependent on family caregivers for self-care Perseverating negative feelings about her future Avoidance/defiance behaviors Difficulty regulating her emotions Feeling of learned helplessness Low self-esteem
PERFORMANCE PATTERNS	Roles: Caroline identifies as a daughter, sister, student, and friend. Routines: Mother assists in dressing, personal hygiene, breakfast, transferring to wheelchair, and escorting her outside her building for wheelchair bus transportation. Outside of school and regular Sunday church attendance, she reports limited community play/leisure opportunities.	

(continued)

TABLE 10-1 (CONTINUED)

Caroline's Occupational Profile

What client factors do Caroline and her team see as supporting engagement in desired occupations, and what aspects are inhibiting engagement?

	SUPPORTING	INHIBITING
VALUES, BELIEFS, AND SPIRITUALITY	Caroline actively engages in all therapies. Caroline has strong religious beliefs and cultural background. Mother is dedicated to Caroline's lifelong well-being. Caroline is social and eager to engage in peer interactions.	Caroline has low self-esteem. Caroline expresses anxiety about future living and vocational opportunities. Caroline reports her friends do not live in accessible homes or have the adult support for her to visit.
BODY FUNCTIONS	Caroline has good sitting balance within her base of support. Caroline navigates and manages her power wheelchair with minimal safety cues within her home and school environment.	Caroline exhibits spasticity in both her arms. Caroline has fluctuating tone in her trunk and right arm. Caroline is dependent on transfers from and to all surfaces. Caroline demonstrates emotional lability, low frustration tolerance, low self-esteem, and learned helplessness.
BODY STRUCTURES	Caroline exhibits right upper extremity involvement. Scoliosis.	Impacts bimanual activities and seating posture in her wheelchair

What are Caroline's and her team's priorities and desired goals?

OCCUPATIONAL PERFORMANCE	Caroline would like to participate in community events such as going to a football game or watching football at her friends' houses.
PREVENTION	Caroline is interested in learning how to navigate her wheelchair from the school building to the athletic field of the school campus.
HEALTH AND WELLNESS	Maintain health and wellness through improved nutrition, standing program, and wheelchair-accessible sports
QUALITY OF LIFE AND WELL-BEING	Improve self-worth, self-advocacy through positive engagement with her family, school staff, and care manager Caroline states she is willing to engage in problem-solving solutions and establish attainable goals for transition planning and community leisure activities.
PARTICIPATION AND ROLE COMPETENCE	Motivated to participate in school-based occupational therapy services to improve social participation across indoor and outdoor school and community settings
OCCUPATIONAL JUSTICE	Seeking access to case managers and the Office for People With Developmental Disabilities to establish realistic community vocational opportunities

Adapted from American Occupational Therapy Association. (2020). AOTA occupational profile template. https://www.aota.org/-/media/Corporate/Files/Practice/Manage/Documentation/AOTA-Occupational-Profile-Template.pdf

Complementary Models of Practice

Because Caroline presents with limitations in range of motion (ROM) and decreased strength through her trunk and extremities as well as tonal abnormalities, the biomechanical and neurodevelopmental frames of reference (FORs) are a good fit to address her challenges in these domains and have good utility to improve motor function and outcomes. The biomechanical and neurodevelopmental treatment (NDT) FORs are widely used interventions when working with children who have physical impairments with diagnoses including cerebral palsy, Down syndrome, traumatic brain injury, and brachial plexus injuries (Cole & Tufano, 2020). These particular FORs tend to have more biomechanically and neurologic-based constructs as their underlying basis.

Additionally, because of her tonal issues, Caroline presents with difficulty maintaining a sitting position and independently navigating her environment and, because of moderate dysarthria, has decreased fluency and intelligibility of her speech. Because she demonstrates strength in her ability to access and use assistive technology, the Human Activity Assistive Technology (HAAT) model was also selected to address her seating, mobility, and communication needs.

Biomechanical Frame of Reference

The biomechanical FOR guides assessment and intervention when there are deficits in the areas of strength, ROM, or endurance affecting the ability to engage in occupations (Cole & Tufano, 2020). As discussed in Chapter 6, this FOR draws heavily on concepts from anatomy, physiology, and kinesiology. Typical assessments used include manual muscle testing, sensation testing, and assessment of ROM. Interventions typically address improving ROM to allow the individual to access or manipulate items in their environment, increase strength to allow for the access or manipulation of objects within and against gravity, and improve endurance to allow individuals to increase their level of effort or time engaged within physical activity (Colangelo & Shea, 2020).

The biomechanical FOR primarily addresses components found in the domains of client factors (body functions and structures) and performance skills (motor skills). "Client factors are affected by occupations, contexts, performance patterns, and performance skills" (AOTA, 2020, p. 15). Client factors of body structures and body functions support students' ability to complete basic motor functions and potentially impact the ability to use the limbs and coordinate the body to participate in all occupations within the educational setting. Using this FOR, a practitioner would observe and assess physical components such as active ROM, strength, and endurance. Both dynamic and static abilities also fall within a biomechanical approach; therefore, practitioners must not only assess a student's ability to move within the school environment but must also assess the student's ability to maintain positions in space. This most notably may be a consideration when observing or assessing a student's ability to sit for prolonged periods of time within a classroom for instruction, to watch a sporting event, or enjoy time with peers at the lunch table.

Primary interventions using a biomechanical FOR typically belong to the area of preparatory methods. The *OTPF-4* identifies preparatory methods as occupational therapy interventions that prepare an individual for "occupational performance, used as part of a treatment session in preparation for or concurrently with occupations and activities ... to support daily occupational performance" (AOTA, 2014, p. S29). Interventions within the preparatory methods appropriate for the school-based setting would include exercise programs to improve ROM, strength, or endurance; seating and positioning modifications; and, if appropriate to the school setting, splint fabrication. When using a biomechanical FOR, practitioners would place focus on addressing how a student is able to access and manipulate objects as well as maintain positions or negotiate their environment for participation. Practitioners need to be mindful when clinically reasoning and treatment planning to keep occupation at the forefront of their decisions in how the improvement in biomechanics improves function in desired school-based occupations. For example, improving hand strength and endurance may be needed for a student to engage in prolonged writing tasks to complete essays on tests.

While assessing Caroline's barriers to participation from a biomechanical perspective, the following were noted:

- Her ability to move both arms through space and against gravity and maintain her position within space is significantly compromised because of spasticity and fluctuating tone.
- She presents with severe lumbar extension (lordosis). She underwent a right femoral hip rotation surgery, which contributed to her asymmetrical sitting posture.
- Caroline is unable to laterally shift her weight over her hips, limiting her lateral and posterior reach beyond arm's length, or initiate sit-to-stand transfers, affecting her ability to obtain and manipulate desired objects in her environment.
- She has limited passive ROM in her lower trunk and lower extremities and lacks trunk rotation, impacting her ability to maintain a seated position, which necessitates adaptive seating in order for her to participate in her school day for academics as well as more leisure-type school activities such as sitting at the lunch table or when spending time with peers at recess.
- She has full passive ROM in both arms; full active ROM in her left shoulder, arm, wrist, and hand; and limited active ROM in her right shoulder, arm, wrist, and hand. Her active ROM deficits make bilateral activities challenging and affect her ability to engage in leisure or play activities.

For Caroline, the use of this FOR as part of intervention includes the use of a right functional hand splint to assist in bimanual activities and a bilateral ankle-foot orthosis through the school day to assist in support during stand pivot transfers and the use of her power wheelchair. Her wheelchair has an elevating seat that raises 12 inches in height to assist in environmental access and face-to-face communication with her peers. She is on a tilt-in-space schedule to reduce sacral pressure but is noncompliant because of peer pressure. Caroline is a skilled power wheelchair user. She is independent in managing all her wheelchair features, except for her foot plates and buckling her seat belt.

Neurodevelopmental Treatment Frame of Reference

NDT has been primarily used as an FOR to address an individual's needs when there are neurologic deficits causing a change in physiological muscle tone throughout the body (Barthel, 2020). Diagnoses with neurologic deficits resulting in tonal abnormalities such as cerebral palsy, Down syndrome, and traumatic brain injury are more typical within the pediatric population and, therefore, school-based settings. Primary *OTPF-4* domains of NDT focus on client factors and performance skills.

The main tenet of NDT lies in the understanding of typical development and movement patterns as a foundation for understanding how the posture and movement systems are integrated within typically developing individuals (Barthel, 2020; Bierman et al., 2016). Impairments of the postural and movement systems are typically found in individuals with cerebral palsy, traumatic brain injuries, or cerebral vascular accidents. Secondary impairments are described as the result of lifelong progression of living with neuromotor impairments with minimal intervention that impact the person's body structures and function in their daily lives. NDT recognizes the dynamics of plasticity, recovery, and compensations throughout the life span within the individual's environmental and personal factors (Bierman et al., 2016).

NDT is a clinically based practice model that relies on current neuroscience and musculoskeletal theories to explain its therapeutic intervention. The primary treatment modality used when applying an NDT FOR is therapeutic handling whereby the practitioner facilitates the essential movement components with environmental and task modification required for optimal task efficiency. In Caroline's case, the optimal goal would be to enhance her participation in play and leisure activities by modifying the task and environmental demands while therapeutically facilitating the movement components needed for the desired play and leisure activity (Barthel, 2020; Bierman et al., 2016). The in-depth understanding of biomechanical alignment and atypical/typical movement patterns across the life span is the foundation for observing, analyzing, and facilitating posture and movement needed for functional tasks.

Caroline desires to increase her ability to participate in play and leisure activities with her family and peers across settings. Caroline expresses frustration over her movement impairment, which affects her level of independence. Her increased and fluctuating tone affects her ability to move, especially her right upper extremity, in typical movement patterns. This impacts her ability to engage in uni- and bilateral activities. She lacks dynamic sitting balance, which causes difficulty in freeing her right upper extremity for bimanual activities, such as art, wheelchair adaptive sports, and personal hygiene. Varying the environment while engaging in desired play and leisure activities will increase her motor planning and motor learning opportunities for motor efficiency and skill acquisition.

Human Activity Assistive Technology Model

When clinically reasoning Caroline's occupational profile in conjunction with her desired participation in play and leisure activities, the HAAT model was also selected to address mobility and communication. The HAAT model describes a framework for identifying a need and place for assistive technology as a means of enhancing the participation and performance in daily life occupations in individuals with disabilities across settings and their life span (Cook & Polgar, 2015). The HAAT has four main components to consider when recommending assistive technology: the human component, the activity component, the assistive technology component, and the contextual component with assistive technology as a separate element as a contributing factor for occupational engagement in daily tasks (Cook & Polgar, 2015).

The human component identifies the individual's physical, cognitive, and emotional factors impacting the daily occupations. For Caroline, there are significant motoric barriers affecting performance including her decreased passive and active ROM, fluctuating muscle tone, musculoskeletal asymmetries, decreased postural strength and endurance, volitional control, motor efficiency, and bimanual manipulation. Cognitive factors affecting performance include her varied levels of arousal, decreased working memory, spatial relations, and difficulty with generalization of skill. Caroline's emotional factors impacting her participation in play and leisure tasks include emotional lability, low self-esteem, and depression and anxiety.

Activity is the fundamental component of the HAAT model and is defined as the act of doing something that represents the outcome of human performance (Cook & Polgar, 2015). The activity represents the individual's occupational competency. Activity categories include activities of daily living, productive activity, work, play, and leisure. The HAAT model breaks down the components of play and leisure to include activities of self-expression, enjoyment, and relaxation. It is the individual's identification of meaning toward that activity that determines its categorization. For example, cooking for one person may be categorized as a productive activity and leisure for another. Activity performance is also influenced by the roles of the temporal and spatial roles of that individual. Cooking for a chef at an upscale restaurant will also differ from the same chef making Sunday breakfast for the family. Additionally, individuals have multiple roles in their daily lives and across their life span.

When assessing activity for Caroline, it is important to define the level of assistance from others for self-care use of assistive technology. Caroline is particular in accepting assistance from others during toileting, impacting community leisure activities with her peers, such as attending high school football games and socializing at her friends' homes or parties. Caroline accepts self-care assistance at her church events because there are familiar adults available within her church community.

The assistive technology component is the interface between the human, the user of the technology, and the device that assists the human in task completion. The assistive technology device is the vehicle for occupational engagement, and modification allows for occupational adaptation (Cook & Polgar, 2015). Caroline's use of assistive technology includes the seating system of her power wheelchair and her augmentative and alternative communication (AAC) device. Caroline has an active role in determining the use of her assistive technology across settings. For example, Caroline's use of her iPad (Apple), which is mounted on her power wheelchair, is dependent on the activity and environmental context. Her iPad functions as an AAC device when she is in crowded or noisy environments such as at recess or in the cafeteria. She presents with moderate dysarthria, demonstrating limited utterances per breath, making her intelligibility difficult for unfamiliar individuals, especially in noisy environments such as the school cafeteria or sporting events. Caroline chooses to use her iPad as an AAC device under these circumstances for increased participation in communication with her peers.

The context is the integration of the human, the activity, and the assistive technology. The context includes the physical context (natural and built environmental factors); social context with familiar and unfamiliar individuals; cultural context; and institutional context (Cook & Polgar, 2015), such as Caroline's school, church, and legal or medical institutions. The context is an essential factor in the individual's efficient use of assistive technology. Contextual factors may provide both supports and barriers for assistive technology efficiency. The user's familiarity within the context is identified as a contributing factor for assistive technology mastery. Caroline's familiarity with managing and navigating her wheelchair in her school setting differs from unfamiliar or novel community settings, such as movie theaters, shopping malls, supermarkets, and churches. Mastery of assistive technology in the school setting may not transfer to mastery of assistive technology in novel settings with unfamiliar variables. Factors such as the level of assistance from others as well as the user skill of the assistive technology (e.g., navigating her power wheelchair up steep hills, ramps, crowded public hallways) impact her occupational competence across settings.

Goals and Interventions

Because person-directed goal setting is an essential component of the OAM (the organizing model of practice in this case), the therapist works with Caroline to determine what types of goals and occupations she wishes to engage in as part of her play and leisure goals. In addition to using the OAM to guide goal development, it is essential to use desired occupations as to how intervention occurs to allow for reflection and assessment of overall satisfaction with performance. It also provides opportunities for modifications or adaptations while performing desired occupations. Based on her current occupational profile and her stated desires, goals for Caroline to address her desired participation in play and leisure include the following:

- The use of an AAC device to engage in conversation with peers during social times such as lunch and recess
- Attending school football games using her chair to navigate the school grounds
- Identifying and engaging in at least one new area of leisure/play based on her areas of personal interest

When using the organizing model of occupational adaptation in conjunction with the complementary models selected of biomechanical, NDT, and HAAT, several approaches to intervention are deemed appropriate to address Caroline's goals. Because Caroline identifies she is dissatisfied with her performance in the area of play and leisure primarily based on her perception that she is limited in her movement and mobility, approaches addressing the ability to establish and restore will address these barriers by promoting improved active ROM and the use of efficient movement patterns via therapeutic handling and exercise as per the biomechanical and NDT FORs. Likewise, using a modification approach, the biomechanical FOR supports the use of splints and her powered chair to maintain proper alignment to be able to engage in activities as well as negotiate her environment. In conjunction with the biomechanical approach, the HAAT model supports the use of the assistive devices to enhance mobility and communication abilities. As per the organizing model, as Caroline engages in her desired occupations, probing her level of satisfaction with her performance can work to enhance her occupational adaptation and allow her to make changes in her strategies to further enhance her satisfaction in occupational participation.

CONCLUSION

In this chapter, we examined how theoretical approaches can be used as a foundation to build person-centered interventions to address the ability to meaningfully engage in play and leisure activities within the school setting. By using an organizing model of practice that capitalized on Caroline's strengths, the intervention was able to address her overall desires and satisfaction with her ability to participate in desired play and leisure activities while addressing her motoric challenges via various complementary models supporting her seating, mobility, and communication needs. In the next chapter, we examine the related occupational area of social participation and how these needs can be addressed within the context of the school setting.

REFERENCES

American Occupational Therapy Association. (2011). Building play skills for healthy children and families. https://www.smallstepsbigleapsnyc.com/wp-content/uploads/2012/02/Play-Skills-Tip-sheet.pdf

American Occupational Therapy Association (2014). Occupational therapy practice framework: Domain and process (3rd Ed.). *American Journal of Occupational Therapy, 68*(Supplement_1), S1-S48. https://doi.org/10.5014/ajot.2014.682006

American Occupational Therapy Association. (2020). Occupational therapy practice framework: Domain and process (4th ed.). *American Journal of Occupational Therapy, 74*(Suppl. 2), 7412410010p1-7412410010p87. https://doi.org/10.5014/ajot.2020.74S2001

Barthel, K. A. (2020). A frame of reference for neuro-developmental treatment. In P. Kramer, J. Hinojosa, & T. H. Howe (Eds.), *Frames of reference for pediatric occupational therapy* (4th ed., pp. 205-246). Wolters Kluwer.

Bierman, J. C., Franjoine, M. R., Hazzard, C. M., Howle, J. M., & Stamer, M. H. (2016). *Neuro-developmental treatment: A guide to NDT clinical practice.* Thieme.

Cahill, S. M., & Beisbier, S. (2020). Practice guidelines—Occupational therapy practice guidelines for children and youth ages 5-21 years. *American Journal of Occupational Therapy, 74,* 7404397010. https://doi.org/10.5014/ajot.2020.744001

Colangelo, C. A., & Shea, M. (2020). A biomechanical frame of reference for positioning children for functioning. In P. Kramer, J. Hinojosa, & T. H. Howe (Eds.), *Frames of reference for pediatric occupational therapy* (4th ed., pp. 247-318). Wolters Kluwer.

Cole, M., & Tufano, R. (2020). *Applied theories in occupational therapy* (2nd ed.). SLACK Incorporated.

Cook, A. M., & Polgar, J. M. (Eds.). (2015). *Assistive technologies: Principles and practice* (4th ed.). Mosby.

Graco, L. (2017). Occupational adaptation. In J. Hinojosa, P. Kramer, & C. Brasic Royeen (Eds.), *Perspectives on human occupation: Theories underlying practice* (2nd ed., pp. 287-312). F. A. Davis.

Parham, L. D., & Fazio, L. S. (Eds.). (1997). *Play in occupational therapy for children.* Mosby.

Parham, L. D., & Fazio, L. (2008). *Play in occupational therapy for children* (2nd ed.). Elsevier.

Schkade, J. K., & Schultz, S. (1992). Occupational adaptation: Toward a holistic approach to contemporary practice, Part 1. *American Journal of Occupational Therapy, 46(9),* 829-837.

11

Social Participation

Miranda Virone, OTD, OTR/L

Chapter Objectives

1. Define the occupation of social participation and describe the ways in which this occupation is experienced in school by students.
2. Identify the ways in which a student's social participation aligns with the purpose and requirements of public school education and its long-term purpose of productive adulthood.
3. Describe the ways in which occupational therapy practitioners evaluate and establish theory-based intervention plans for students with needs in the area of social participation and interdependence.

Human beings are innately social beings. Our ability to connect and interact with others is a biological predisposition necessary for survival that is hardwired in our neurologic system (Cook, 2013). The work of anthropologists, psychologists, and other social scientists explores various theories that describe the significant impact social connectivity has on cognitive, physical, and emotional development. Our ability to form a bond with a parent, trust among friends, and intimacy with a partner is tied to early social experiences (Goren et al., 1975). To the contrary, these scientists also identify the harmful and damaging effects delayed, limited, or complete absence of social interaction can have on the typical development of humans. Intellectual disability, mental illness, and predisposition to a number of diseases can all manifest as a result of limited, unhealthy, or a lack of social opportunities (Hawkley & Cacioppo, 2010).

Laverdure, P., & Seruya, F. M. *Theory in School-Based Occupational Therapy Practice: A Practical Application* (pp. 147-163). DOI: 10.4324/9781003526773-11

Occupational scientists further explore the potential injustices that can result from disrupted or narrowed social experiences using an occupational justice lens. Social deprivation, imbalance, alienation, and marginalization can impact the degree to which humans participate socially. Exclusion, rejection, and being alienated or ostracized from social experiences impact participation in a vital occupation and can therefore disrupt overall health and well-being (Kronenberg & Pollard, 2006).

Social participation is one of nine areas of occupation identified by the fourth edition of the *Occupational Therapy Practice Framework: Domain and Process* published by the American Occupational Therapy Association (AOTA, 2020b). Social participation is described as activities that involve social interaction with others, including family, friends, peers, and community members, and that support social interdependence (AOTA, 2020b, p. 34; Bedell, 2012; Khetani & Coster, 2019; Magasi & Hammel, 2004). The framework identifies five components of social participation: community participation, family participation, friendships, intimate partner relationships, and peer group interaction. Social participation is strongly influenced by other aspects of the practice framework domains including performance patterns, performance skills, client factors, and contexts. Contexts involve environmental and personal factors that may impact access to occupations and the ability to satisfactorily engage in occupations (World Health Organization, 2008).

SOCIAL PARTICIPATION IN THE SCHOOL CONTEXT

Environmental and Personal Factors

School, as a context for social participation, offers a unique set of environmental and personal factors for students. Environmental factors that can impact social participation may include technology; support/relationships; attitudes; and services, systems, and policies. These factors "can either enable or restrict participation in meaningful occupations and can present barriers to or supports and resources for service delivery" (AOTA, 2020b, p. 10). Personal factors that can influence social participation in the school context include age, sexual orientation, sex/race/cultural identity, socioeconomic status, upbringing, behavior, personality traits, lifestyle, and health conditions. Students in the school context often have shared or similar personal factors that can contribute to the formation of groups, a dynamic that has the capacity to enhance or complicate social participation. Environmental and personal factors of social participation in the school context can be further explored in subcontexts that consist of school transportation, the classroom, the cafeteria, recess, and extracurricular activities.

School Transportation

The school bus offers a unique set of environmental and personal factors pertaining to social participation. The environmental factors of a school bus involve limited structure and direct supervision of students, with a ratio of one adult to an entire bus full of students. This common scenario lends itself to opportunities for students to demonstrate and communicate a variety of personal factors among their peers. Personal factors such as behavior, lifestyle, personality characteristics, and social status can all be conveyed through actions, verbal conversation, or device use via text or social media. Personal factors are also key components on how one student or a group of peers respond and interact with others in this unstructured subcontext of the school bus. Negative interactions are more likely to occur as a result.

Classroom

The classroom offers a number of social participation opportunities for students with greater levels of structure and support from the teacher and school. Students interact individually and within peer groups to complete academic tasks but are also engaging socially where personal factors become involved. Most social interaction in the classroom occurs with verbal interaction and can be moderated by the teacher to remain positive and healthy. The vast reality is that many schools do allow personal cell phones in middle and high school grade levels (and occasionally even elementary grade levels). This creates an opportunity for unstructured social interaction where content cannot necessarily be monitored.

Cafeteria

The school cafeteria is a place known for robust social interaction. Students enter the cafeteria with excitement to escape academic tasks, and most are eager to engage with their peers. Structure is nominal. Supervision is available but indirect. Conversation is free flowing. The cafeteria is where many students are more relaxed to be themselves among their peers and can enjoy personal conversation. The cafeteria can also be a daunting place for some students. Loud voices, busy bodies, and exclusive peer groups can deter those students from social interaction.

Recess

Recess is a more notable time for social participation at school. It is another opportunity to engage with peers and to move a body that has been seated for much of the day. Recess can have varying degrees of environmental structure and support based on who is monitoring, the physical equipment and space available, and the types of activities that are available. Students can interact one to one or in peer groups freely. The environmental factors will strongly influence the dynamics of student personal factors related to positive peer interaction. Limited structure and support may result in more student creativity but also more peer conflict. Excess structure and support may result in limited social participation opportunities but no conflict. This may result in an occupational imbalance. A balance of both can create a number of healthy social experiences during recess.

Extracurricular Activities

School-supported extracurricular activities are an incredible way to offer students more opportunities to be involved in tasks they enjoy and can participate in socially. Extracurricular activities are often chosen specifically by the student based on their desire to engage in a certain type of task. This is generally a shared personal interest or factor among peer groups. Environmental support and structure can vary based on the age of the student, the type of activity, and the number of adults involved. However, it is important to consider social participation injustices that can result from extracurricular activities that are not accessible to students because of academic ineligibility, the costs involved, or disability. Policy consideration, financial support, and accommodations must be involved to create an equitable opportunity for all students to participate in these socially meaningful experiences.

CASE STUDY

Maggie is a 16-year-old female student in ninth grade who attends a suburban public high school with a population of approximately 135 students per grade level. Academically, Maggie is an average to above average student who particularly enjoys academic electives such as band, chorus, and visual arts. Her most challenging subjects include history and algebra, which require her to attend in-school tutoring sessions for extra academic support. Maggie participates in extracurricular activities such as marching band, school musicals, Pride Club, and track and field. She reports having two to three close friends at school with whom she socializes with in class, in the cafeteria, and via text messaging. Maggie has experienced intermittent bullying based on the sexual orientation of her friends and herself.

Maggie lives with her mother, stepfather, and 8-year-old sister in an upper, middle-class neighborhood. She has a close relationship with her mother with whom she feels comfortable talking to about personal issues in most instances. Maggie recently shared with her mother that she identifies as pansexual. Maggie's relationship with her stepfather has had challenges in the past regarding behaviors she displayed of which he did not approve. These included her disinterest in participating in chores, excessive screen time use, and disrespectful language and actions aimed at her mother. In recent years, these behaviors have declined, and her relationship with her stepfather has improved. Maggie's interaction with her younger sister is mostly positive. The 7-year age difference creates challenges in finding similar interests and activities they both enjoy together. They occasionally argue when her younger sister wants to play, but Maggie is not interested in the chosen activity. Maggie's preferred activities at home include playing games on her phone, painting her nails, putting on makeup, and occasionally drawing or reading. Drawing and reading were preferred activities of hers before receiving a smartphone in eighth grade. She has had friendships with other children in her neighborhood in the past but no longer actively pursues activities with them. She does enjoy connecting with two to three friends for social activities outside of school, but these occasions are typically facilitated by her mother.

Maggie was diagnosed with combined type attention-deficit/hyperactivity disorder (ADHD) and generalized anxiety disorder (GAD) at age 10 years. ADHD is characterized by deficits in executive function skills that persist for 6 months or more (American Psychiatric Association, 2013). Maggie's ADHD symptoms include inattentiveness, impulsivity, emotional dysregulation, impaired planning and organization, and impaired metacognition skills. GAD is diagnosed when excessive worry occurs more often than not throughout a 6-month time frame and impairs key areas of function (American Psychiatric Association, 2013). Maggie's GAD symptoms include excessive worry that impairs her ability to enjoy pleasurable activities. Maggie is prescribed methylphenidate and sertraline to manage her ADHD and GAD symptoms. Recently, Maggie began experiencing increased feelings of hopelessness and loneliness that persisted and affected her daily participation in occupations. She was subsequently diagnosed with depression. Her neuropsychologist increased her sertraline dosage to manage these new symptoms.

Maggie receives counseling services on an outpatient basis intermittently when symptoms escalate, new symptoms arise, or when medication changes occur. She also visits with the school counselor when she feels challenged by her symptoms at school or when social interactions become too complex for her to manage independently. The combination of interventions has been positive, but she continues to struggle with making new friends and sustaining healthy friendships. Table 11-1 provides an analysis of Maggies's occupational profile.

TABLE 11-1

Maggie's Occupational Profile

What concerns do Maggie and her team have about her occupational engagement?	Maggie was referred to occupational therapy for concerns expressed by several of her teachers that she rarely engages with other students, is frequently distracted by her personal phone, and does not appear to enjoy once-preferred classes. Maggie's band teacher expressed concerns that Maggie rarely engages in conversation with students she previously was known to be friends with within her instrument section. He is concerned about Maggie's withdrawn behavior and recent disinterest in band. Maggie's English teacher reports Maggie does not engage with peers during group activities. She is often distracted in groups by her phone and has been asked repeatedly to put it away. Maggie replies to the request but pulls the phone out of her pocket any time a notification alert is heard. Her teacher is concerned that Maggie is missing key interactions due to the frequent phone distractions. She reports this has resulted in her below average grade in English. Maggie's visual arts teacher noted that Maggie does not engage in effective social interaction with the teacher or other students. She often seems disinterested and disengaged. She replies to questions from the teacher and peers with brief answers and flat emotion. Maggie does not initiate contributions to class discussion and is often seen scrolling through her computer rather than attending to the topic being taught. Maggie's teacher is concerned about her lack of interest in a class she was once so enthusiastic about.
In what occupations is Maggie successful, and what barriers impact her success?	Maggie is a talented artist. She has attended private art classes in the past and won various awards for her artwork. She is especially skilled in anime drawings, landscape painting, and charcoal sketching. Maggie also is an incredible musician with the guitar, vocals, saxophone, and clarinet. She takes private guitar and voice lessons and is in the marching band where she plays saxophone, the school band where she plays clarinet, and school musicals where she performs in the vocal ensemble. She struggles with social interactions as a result of her ADHD and anxiety symptoms. She is known to be impulsive with her thoughts becoming words that may not be appropriate for the timing or content of conversation with others. This has resulted in her unknowingly offending others or being perceived as odd. Her self-awareness of these symptoms and factors has grown in recent years and has resulted in social anxiety that prevents her from freely engaging in peer conversation for fear she will embarrass herself or inadvertently offend someone. Maggie has become socially withdrawn and prefers to engage with her phone as a substitute for anxiety-producing, face-to-face, social interaction.

(continued)

TABLE 11-1 (CONTINUED)
Maggie's Occupational Profile

What is Maggie's occupational history?	Maggie attended a private, faith-based school from preschool through fourth grade until her parents divorced. When her mother remarried, the family moved, and Maggie transitioned into public school for fifth grade. Maggie quickly made friends and would frequently be invited to parties and sleepovers. The following year, she and her group of friends transitioned to sixth grade in the middle school building. Her group of friends slowly declined because classes did not have the same group of students. Many of her previous friends formed or joined cliques that Maggie was not welcomed into or did not feel she belonged to. She continued to maintain a connection with three to five friends with whom she would sit with at lunch and would invite her to events. By the end of eighth grade, the final year of middle school, Maggie maintained friendships with two other students who she continued to sit with at lunch. However, invitations for sleepovers and events waned, and Maggie's mother began reaching out to the parents of those two friends to invite them for sleepovers or to movies. By ninth grade, Maggie reported having one close friend who identified as bisexual and nonbinary and was frequently harassed and bullied by other students.
What are Maggie's and her team's personal interests and values?	Maggie values her relationship with her family and enjoys watching movies, playing games, and traveling with them. She also values her few friendships and activities she participates in at school. Maggie is interested in art and wishes to pursue a degree in digital graphic design. She enjoys playing games on her phone and using art apps on her phone to color and draw. Maggie's interests also include singing and playing musical instruments.
What aspects of the contexts do Maggie and her team see as supporting engagement in desired occupations, and what aspects are inhibiting engagement?	
ENVIRONMENT	Maggie lives with her mother, stepfather, younger sister, cat, and dog in a two-story home located in a suburban neighborhood. Her parents are both teachers who value education and family values. They are Christians who occasionally attend church. Maggie attends the local public high school with other students in Grades 9 through 12. The school consists of predominantly White, middle-class students. Various support services are available including guidance counseling, counseling psychology, and occupational therapy.
PERSONAL	Maggie is 16 years old, White, female, and pansexual. She comes from a middle-class, working family that consists of her, her mother, her stepfather, and her younger sister. Maggie is diagnosed with ADHD, GAD, and depression and uses prescribed medication to manage her symptoms. She can become easily stressed with multiple demands or responsibilities, when she is asked to do something she does not want to do, or when she is asked to put her phone down to engage in another task.

(continued)

TABLE 11-1 (CONTINUED)
Maggie's Occupational Profile

PERFORMANCE PATTERNS	This portion of the occupational profile will explore Maggie's patterns of engagement in occupation, how they have changed in recent months, and what her daily life roles involve (AOTA, 2020b). Maggie is most productive and efficient with a set routine. Her weekday morning routine is consistent and rarely changes. She wakes, gets dressed, eats breakfast, brushes her teeth and hair, gathers her coat and backpack, and then heads out to the bus. Her daily schedule at school only varies quarterly. Her afternoon routine changes based on the extracurricular activity she is engaged in. The after-school time frame is the most inconsistent in her day and can cause problems with remembering schedules or forgetting needed items. Maggie's primary roles include daughter, sister, and student with mental health diagnoses.
What client factors do Maggie and her team see as supporting engagement in desired occupations, and what aspects are inhibiting engagement?	
VALUES, BELIEFS, AND SPIRITUALITY	Maggie values time to herself and engaging in preferred, personally motivating activities such as playing games or using art applications (apps) on her phone while alone in her bedroom. She believes she should not have screen time or content limits and should be trusted to use her phone as she wishes. Maggie also values activities with her family when it suits her. She values friends who allow her to feel she can be herself by speaking freely and openly.
BODY FUNCTIONS	Maggie struggles with specific mental functions involving attention, working memory, and emotion. These challenges are congruent with the executive function deficits that are characteristic symptoms associated with her ADHD diagnosis. She also has difficulty with global mental functions involving psychosocial, temperament, and personality characteristics necessary for positive social interactions. She struggles with motivation for nonpreferred and occasionally preferred activities. The factors may be more closely related to her GAD and depression diagnoses.
BODY STRUCTURES	Maggie's diagnosis of ADHD indicates neurodiversity or changes in the neurologic system most notably found in the limbic system and prefrontal cortex. These areas are associated with self-regulation and higher-level executive function skills. Abnormalities in these neurologic structures are common in adolescents with ADHD (Barkley, 2015).

(continued)

TABLE 11-1 (CONTINUED)	
Maggie's Occupational Profile	
What are Maggie's and her team's priorities and desired goals?	
OCCUPATIONAL PERFORMANCE	Maggie wishes to perform better academically and socially. She wants to feel confident and competent as a student and peer for successful performance in education and social participation. Maggie expresses a desire to feel more comfortable when surrounded by peers. She would like to freely contribute to conversation without fear of saying something wrong or offending others. Maggie wishes others knew how hard it is for her to talk to others and express herself without anxiety. She wants to enjoy art class without worrying, and she wishes she felt accepted by more than just one or two friends. Maggie reports she wants very much to feel included and belong to a group of peers.
PREVENTION	Maggie's desire is that her symptoms and challenges no longer impede her occupational performance. She hopes occupational therapy interventions will prevent further symptom development that can impact occupational performance
HEALTH AND WELLNESS	Maggie's priority is to manage her anxiety, depression, and mental health symptoms discreetly, effectively, and as independently as possible. She desires to be mentally healthy and agrees she needs support to achieve this outcome.
QUALITY OF LIFE AND WELL-BEING	Maggie desires to feel joy and happiness throughout her daily activities. She wishes she did not have intense episodes of loneliness and sadness that impair her ability to enjoy tasks that typically appeal to her.
PARTICIPATION AND ROLE COMPETENCE	Maggie's priority is to be a good daughter, sister, student, and friend. It is important to her that others view her in this way and that she feels confident and competent in her roles.
OCCUPATIONAL JUSTICE	Maggie has experienced occupational deprivation in the school environment while being socially excluded by peers. Social exclusion has limited her opportunities for social participation and the formation of meaningful connections with peers. Lack of meaningful peer relationships can directly impact health, well-being, and quality of life (Holt-Lunstad et al., 2010).

Adapted from American Occupational Therapy Association. (2020a). AOTA occupational profile template. https://www.aota.org/-/media/Corporate/Files/Practice/Manage/Documentation/AOTA-Occupational-Profile-Template.pdf

Organizing Model of Practice:
Model of Human Occupation

The Model of Human Occupation (MOHO) will serve as the organizing model of practice (OMP) to guide the occupational therapist through assessment, goal development, and intervention planning in Maggie's case (Ikiugu et al., 2009). MOHO was developed by Gary Kielhofner based on the work of Mary Reilly's occupational behavior theory. Kielhofner aimed to develop a systems-based model that could offer a holistic approach to occupational engagement across the life span. MOHO is centered around the importance of occupation and involves four key elements: volition, habituation, performance capacity, and environment (Cole & Tufano, 2020). Disruption in any element of the system causes a shift or disturbance in the client's pattern of behavior signaling the need for change. Occupational therapy practitioners who use MOHO as an OMP help clients recognize changes in occupational performance and assist with developing new patterns of performance through evaluation, intervention, and outcome measures. MOHO has been applied and researched internationally to various populations, ages, and abilities with convincing evidence to support its efficacy as a conceptual practice model (Taylor, 2017).

Model of Human Occupation Construct

The four key elements of MOHO interact dynamically and reciprocally as a person engages in occupation. Volition involves motivating factors in the client's life. Motivating factors may include values, personal causation, and interests (i.e., what the client feels is important, what they feel they are capable of doing, and what they find enjoyable; Taylor, 2017). Volition is heavily influenced by personal factors including culture, social background, and life experiences. Changes in personal factors may alter what the client feels is important and enjoyable.

Example: Two 15-year-old students were best friends from ages 9 to 12 years. One of the friends has become involved in other school activities and no longer interacts with the other. This may change the value of the school and social experience for the other student.

Habituation describes the patterns, roles, and routines of daily occupations (Taylor, 2017). Environmental factors such as natural events, time-related changes, and technology strongly influence habits and roles. Changes in environmental factors can easily impact our patterns of behavior, causing disruption in a system that was once stable and predictable.

Example: A student is given a Chromebook to take notes on in class instead of using pencil and paper. This technology change may impact the way information is processed during class time.

Performance capacity refers to the physical and mental abilities required for the client to engage in occupations (Cole & Tufano, 2020).

Motor, process, and social skills are goal-directed actions that allow the client to perform occupations with desired outcome quality (AOTA, 2020b). Impaired performance skills can negatively impact performance capacity.

Example: A student may experience symptoms of social anxiety that prevent them from initiating conversation with peers. This may impact performance in social contexts.

The environment also influences participation when considering physical, occupational, and social components and qualities. Changes in environmental components or quality can impact motivation, organization, or participation (Taylor, 2017).

Example: A teacher may choose to move desks apart in a classroom to prevent copying or cheating on work. This environmental change can impact social interactions among students.

Occupational therapy practitioners use MOHO to inform the occupational therapy process when disruption occurs. Interventions are designed to address volition, habituation, and performance capacities that are strongly influenced by the client's environmental and personal factors.

Model of Human Occupation Application

In the case of Maggie, MOHO is the primary OMP. Maggie is struggling with social participation at school. Her teachers report that she is withdrawn during class time and does not engage with peers as she once did. They also report she is frequently distracted by her cell phone and Chromebook. The occupational profile indicates that Maggie's interests, or volition, include art, music, and spending time with her two friends and family. Habituation includes her patterns of behavior, roles, and routines. This has changed significantly with the increased amount of time she spends on her phone or computer while at school. Performance capacity is impacted by executive function/process skill delays that impede Maggie's ability to self-monitor screen time and appropriateness of social behavior. Environmental factors in occupational and social components have changed with more technology-based assignments and decreased friendships and support at school.

Maggie has experienced disturbances in various aspects of a dynamic system. These disturbances have negatively affected social participation in the school environment. Maggie has identified the desire to feel more comfortable around her peers, have more friendships, and communicate without anxiety. Her desire to change is present; however, she does not understand how to orchestrate change. Thus, she relies more heavily on comfortable patterns and habits such as phone and computer use at school to avoid making changes that challenge her performance capacities and executive function skills. MOHO offers a conceptual guide to transforming Maggie's thoughts, feelings, and doings of social participation. Lasting change and new balance for her social participation can be achieved in a supportive and consistent environment (O'Brien & Kielhofner, 2017).

Occupation-Based Evaluation

Occupational therapy will use MOHO and explore other conceptual models of practice to complete the occupational therapy process. Maggie has several strengths in the form of talents and interests. Her love for music and art has continued despite the recent disruption in social participation. Maggie participates in several extracurricular activities during and after the school day. Her family is present, supportive, and involved in her mental health care. Maggie also has one or two close friends she is comfortable being herself around and confiding in. Her teachers are concerned and supportive of her overall health and well-being as indicated by their reports and referral for occupational therapy services.

Maggie has experienced an exacerbation of her anxiety symptoms that combined with her executive function challenges has caused a decline in social participation while at school. Initiating and contributing to group conversation with peers causes increased anxiety. The integration of additional technology use in the school environment has made it convenient for Maggie to disengage in social participation as she shifts her attention to interaction with her smartphone and Chromebook during class time. Furthermore, Maggie has difficulty moderating the impulse to use her phone and monitor time spent on devices because of executive function deficits.

An additional assessment tool supporting the volitional component of MOHO is the Volitional Questionnaire. This assessment will carefully examine motivational elements of Maggie's life. The Volitional Questionnaire is a 14-item questionnaire designed to assess adolescent, adult, and older adult motivation and the environmental impact on occupational participation. The questionnaire requires the rater to observe the client in their natural environment to complete each of the 14 items pertaining to achievement, competency, and exploration along a continuum of sense of ability and control within the environment. The administrator guidelines suggest that Volitional Questionnaire observations take place more than once and in more than one natural environment for the client (De Las Heras et al., 2007).

In the case of Maggie, the Volitional Questionnaire will provide valuable feedback on her level of volitional development. She will be observed while at school during each period where problems were identified—band, algebra, and visual arts. This approach will satisfy more than one observation period and multiple environments as suggested by the questionnaire directions. Item ratings will identify her level of engagement ranging from passive to hesitant to involved to spontaneous while congruently indicating the need for more or less support. The results of the Volitional Questionnaire will guide Maggie's interventions by informing the evaluator on areas of low volition and high support.

Theoretical Appropriateness of the Model of Human Occupation

MOHO most appropriately integrates theory and practice by providing an occupation-based, client-centered approach to Maggie's case that identifies faulty roles and habits disrupting performance capacities while considering areas of occupation that are motivating to her (Ikiugu & Smallfield, 2015). MOHO as the OMP provides an overall lens through which Maggie's occupational performance issues can be understood. Integrating complementary models of practice, or complementary theoretical strategies, through a clinical-reasoning approach will further identify specific assessment tools and intervention strategies to guide the occupational therapy process (Ikiugu, 2012). Collaborative use of a single OMP and one or more complementary models of practice that can change over time offers a dynamic and fluid approach to meeting Maggie's occupational performance needs (Ikiugu et al., 2009). In her case, the occupational therapist will incorporate the Positive Mental Health Framework (PMHF) that can be integrated into the school environment and the social cognitive theory (SCT) to address faulty behavioral processes associated with Maggie's social participation deficits.

Complementary Models of Practice

Positive Mental Health Framework

The PMHF is built on concepts from positive psychology. This model of practice approaches the concept of positive mental health as a foundation for well-being that includes social connectivity. In Maggie's case, mental health and well-being are influenced by social interaction participation and performance. Positive mental health is theoretically rooted in positive psychology, the study of positive mental health aimed to address negative life experiences through building positive qualities such as character strengths and enjoyable experiences (Gable & Haidt, 2005; Seligman, 2002; Seligman & Csikszentmihalyi, 2000). This model of practice encompasses four characteristics that include positive attitudes and emotions, positive mental and social ability, participation in necessary and important activities, and effective coping strategies and resilience (Bazyk, 2020). The promotion of PMHF requires a mindset shift to consider mental health as a necessary aspect of overall health and quality of life that is essential for optimal engagement in occupations in various environments (Barry & Jenkins, 2007).

School Mental Health (SMH) is an interdisciplinary, school-wide approach to mental health promotion and prevention among school-age children and adolescents (Koller & Bertel, 2006; Masia-Warner et al., 2006). SMH initiatives have grown in recent years with the increased prevalence of anxiety, depression, and other mental health disorders that can impact student engagement and performance during the academic day. The addition of social-emotional learning curricula, self-regulation programs, and psychological counseling services has become integral components of school supports offered to students. Various school personnel including administrators, faculty, staff, and related services providers have been recruited to become part of SMH initiatives.

A public health framework or the Multitiered System of Supports (MTSS) is the preferred approach to applying SMH concepts. MTSS is a continuum of care that provides three tiers of supports using a population- and strengths-based approach (Bazyk, 2020). This framework is familiar to public schools because it is used for academic initiatives and is therefore ideal to address SMH initiatives using the same approach. The three tiers of intervention to support mental health promotion and prevention within the MTSS framework include (a) universal or whole-school strategies for everyone; (b) targeted, small-group, embeddable strategies; and (c) intensive, individualized strategies for students experiencing challenges (Bazyk, 2020).

Maggie will benefit from PMHF concepts used within a public health or MTSS framework to address her mental health and social needs at school. Universal strategies that can benefit whole-school positive mental health include faculty professional development focused on PMHF approaches with students, embeddable strategies such as mindfulness to reduce anxiety during social participation, and implementation of mentor or buddy programs to engage students with others. Targeted approaches that may improve social participation for Maggie can include careful observation of social interactions to identify situational stressors, introducing small-group activities with conversation prompts for each group member, and positive self-talk strategies to encourage her during moments of social interaction when she becomes uncomfortable. Intense approaches may include individualized instruction with Maggie on self-regulation techniques such as deep breathing to manage anxiety, collaboration with classroom teachers on embeddable strategies such as a conversation starter that can be used daily to improve social participation, and instructing her to use a journal to document her stressors and the techniques she successfully uses to manage them.

Social Cognitive Theory

SCT is a systems model that considers brain and social development as integral to one another (Bandura, 2001). This model of practice describes cognitive function and social function as innately connected. In Maggie's case, her executive function skills are a component of cognitive function and directly impact her social abilities. SCT suggests that neurologic development and human interaction shape our behavior. Neurologic development of areas of the brain such as the amygdala and prefrontal cortex that are associated with executive function skills can influence social behavior. Human interaction through role participation within social environments allows for learning by observing the actions and responses of others (Adolphs, 2009). For the school-age adolescent, roles may include student, friend, athlete, performer, and so on. Role competence is the perception of which the adolescent believes they successfully fulfill their roles whether individually or within a group. SCT stresses interventions that recognize, integrate, understand, manage, regulate, and express emotions in healthy ways (Mayer et al., 2008).

SCT involves social and emotional reasoning among adolescent clients. Social reasoning explores the important social contexts and occupations that are meaningful to clients. Social reasoning in occupational therapy assumes the following assumptions: roles within social participation are inherent to the occupation and are inseparable, social connectivity impacts occupational choices, social ability impacts the success of social participation, distinct social roles can impact social participation, and effective management of social relationships within contexts can improve social participation (Cole & Tufano, 2020). Social reasoning can influence how connected, motivated, accepted, and involved an adolescent feels in their social environment.

Emotional reasoning consists of the ability to perceive, understand, and regulate emotions and is a product of emotional intelligence, or the ability to problem solve (Mayer & Salovey, 2004). Emotional intelligence encompasses four quadrants of skills: our own perception of emotion, managing our emotions in an acceptable way, our perceptions of others' emotions, and productively managing relationship dynamics (Goleman, 1996). Emotional reasoning influences how an adolescent perceives, manages, and responds to emotional stressors within social contexts.

The disruption in social interaction with Maggie is understood using SCT. Executive dysfunction is a defining symptom of ADHD with neurologic implications in the amygdala and prefrontal cortex, areas of the brain that are critical for social development. Her inability to regulate impulsive speech and behavior receives negative feedback from peer interaction during role participation. Social and emotional reasoning become disrupted through perceptions of role incompetence and emotional stressors that cause her to withdraw from social participation. Healthy emotional perception, management, and expression will be key skills addressed in interventions. Activities such as creative expression projects, reflective journaling, positive affirmations, mindfulness, and a mentoring partner can all contribute to the development of executive function skills and positive peer interaction necessary for improved social participation.

The assessment of Maggie's social and cognitive abilities using an embeddable strategy is most appropriately addressed using the social profile. The social profile is a 26-item observational assessment used to measure levels of cooperation of groups or an individual within an activity group. The social profile was designed based on Mosey's (1986) concept of social interaction and group development principles. The social profile measures social participation using a 26-item profile in a single observation session or across several observation sessions. Three topics identified for assessment include activity participation, social interaction, and group membership and roles. The evaluator uses three levels of group participation including parallel, associative, and basic cooperation to assess the frequency of which behaviors occur (Donahue, 2013). The social profile offers an embeddable assessment approach that can be completed within the school environment using observations that do not disrupt classroom or group dynamics.

The social profile will provide valuable feedback regarding Maggie's social participation within a group activity during band period. The band teacher identified Maggie's lack of initiative and participation during group activities. This environment will provide the evaluator the greatest amount of information using observations guided by the social profile assessment. Item ratings will indicate Maggie's level of frequency of activity participation, social interaction, and group membership and roles during the three levels of group participation. The results of the social profile will identify Maggie's social interaction strengths and challenges during group activities.

Intervention Goals

The following goals were established by Maggie and her team to address her ability to identify, plan, and implement social interaction skills throughout the school day to strengthen peer relationships, self-confidence, and comfort with social interdependence as evidenced through self/teacher report and data collection:

- Maggie will use learned conversation starter strategies to initiate two conversations with two different students in her band section throughout the 38-minute period with no more than one verbal cue from the teacher to improve comfort with in-person social interaction skills as evidenced through band teacher reports and private journaling.
- Maggie will increase the frequency of peer group interaction/reduce the frequency of distraction with a minimum of two, positive verbal contributions to the group process while refraining from phone use during English class (38 minutes) by independently checking her phone into a class phone basket as evidenced by teacher report and a phone check-in/out sheet.
- Maggie will complete a weekly social skills goal-setting worksheet and checklist with assistance/ guidance to identify class contribution and peer group participation strategies for visual arts that include a minimum of three action items to use every day as evidenced by a self-monitored checklist.

Intervention Outcomes

The intervention outcomes in Maggie's case aim to address improvement, health and well-ness, participation, role competence, and well-being. Improvement will result in the adaptation and development of the social and process performance skills that are limited. Health and wellness outcomes will impact self-advocacy skills and empowerment through positive social experiences. Participation will result in personally satisfying social interaction including conversation and in-teraction with peers in various school contexts. Role competence will produce effective skills in the roles of student, friend, and peer. Well-being outcomes will foster a sense of belonging among a peer group, opportunities for self-determination, and overall contentment with life (AOTA, 2020a).

Intervention Plan

Occupational therapy interventions will use three approaches in Maggie's plan: create/promote, establish/restore, and modify. Occupational therapy will develop SMH initiatives using a public health framework to create and promote school-wide positive mental health initiatives at the uni-versal level. These initiatives will include cafeteria and free time strategies for healthy peer engage-ment and fulfilling occupational engagement during mealtime, study time, and social opportuni-ties. Occupational therapy will aim to establish and restore social and process skills for improved confidence during peer interaction. These interventions are reflective of SCT and may include re-flective journaling, positive peer modeling, and role-playing activities to build social skills neces-sary to initiate and sustain conversation, self-regulate impulsive reactions, and monitor social cues. Occupational therapy will implement motivational approaches to modify Maggie's behavior through the use of social strategy checklists, art and music conversation starter tip sheets, and phone check-points that accrue minutes during free periods to spend in small-group activities and games. This approach is consistent with the volition-focused MOHO and will allow Maggie to explore new peer interactions and reduce the amount of social distraction caused by her smartphone (AOTA, 2020a).

Methods for Service Delivery

Occupations and Activities

Social participation and education are meaningful occupations throughout Maggie's life. Using components of these occupations as activities during one-on-one intervention sessions can be ben-eficial when addressing participation and role competence. For example, role-playing and social stories can be used to explore and build social participation preparedness under less stressful cir-cumstances while practicing with the occupational therapist. Maggie can then apply these skills in the classroom context with greater comfort when initiating peer conversation or contributing to classroom conversation.

Education and Training

SMH initiatives require buy-in and support from administration, faculty, and staff members throughout the school. Education and training are essential components of SMH programming. In Maggie's school, the occupational therapist will educate administrators on the vast benefits of school-wide SMH initiatives, provide professional development training to prepare faculty and staff for program implementation, and then function as the program facilitator while coaching faculty and staff to embed strategies throughout the school day. This programming will benefit Maggie by allowing her to experience healthy social opportunities with peers during nonacademic times at school.

Advocacy and Self-Advocacy

Occupational therapy will pursue advocacy efforts that aim to influence school administration perception and understanding of occupational therapy involvement in SMH initiatives. This will include the role of occupational therapy practitioners as specialized instruction support personnel service providers as part of the Every Student Succeeds Act that acknowledges the role of occupational therapy as a member of the multidisciplinary team within the school that can contribute to school programming in various capacities (Bazyk et al., 2022). These programs can benefit students such as Maggie who experience an occupational imbalance involving daily social participation. Occupational therapy will further support Maggie by encouraging her to self-advocate for accommodations such as journaling or consulting with her occupational therapist to ease her anxiety before, during, or after a particularly challenging social experience.

Group Interventions

Maggie will benefit from small social groups organized and facilitated by occupational therapy. Small groups will provide her with an opportunity to gain experience and implement effective social participation strategies in a controlled, supportive, and more comfortable context where her anxiety can be monitored and managed. These facilitated groups will use games and activities beginning with the inclusion of familiar peers and gradually introducing nonfamiliar peers. Group interventions will provide opportunities for meaningful social participation that encourages skill acquisition, self-regulation, and positive choice making using activities such as board games, role-playing, and charades (AOTA, 2020a). Small social groups will allow Maggie to experience social participation competency that can be graded to less facilitation and then generalized into unsupported personal and environmental contexts of the school for successful occupational participation.

Conclusion

Social participation is an integral component of adolescent development. Positive experiences with social participation have the capacity to influence positive mental health and well-being. Adolescents, such as Maggie, can struggle with occupational performance and participation when social skills and abilities do not meet social demand. Establishing a guiding model of practice to identify assessment measures, completing the occupational profile, establishing client-centered goals, and developing meaningful interventions can support positive outcomes. Occupational therapy practitioners can support social participation among adolescents through the use of activities, education and training, advocacy, and group intervention to establish, restore, and maintain occupational performance and participation.

REFERENCES

Adolphs, R. (2009). The social brain: Neural basis of social knowledge. *Annual Review of Psychology, 60*, 693-716.

American Occupational Therapy Association. (2020a). AOTA's occupational profile template: Occupational profile. https://www.aota.org/practice/practice-essentials/documentation/improve-your-documentation-with-aotas-updated-occupational-profile-template

American Occupational Therapy Association. (2020b). Occupational therapy practice framework: Domain and process (4th ed.). *American Journal of Occupational Therapy, 74*(Suppl. 2), 7412410010p1-7412410010p87. https://doi.org/10.5014/ajot.2020.74S2001

American Psychiatric Association. (2013). *Diagnostic and statistical manual of mental health disorders* (5th ed.). American Psychiatric Publishing.

Bandura, A. (2001). Social cognitive theory: An agentic perspective. *Annual Review of Psychology, 52*, 1-26.

Barkley, R. A. (2015). *Attention-deficit hyperactivity disorder: A handbook for diagnosis and Treatment* (4th ed.). Guilford Press.

Barry, M. M., & Jenkins, R. (2007). *Implementing mental health promotion*. Churchill Livingstone/Elsevier.

Bazyk, S. (2020). *Foundations of Every Moment Counts: Positive mental health*. Every Moment Counts. https://s3.us-east-2.amazonaws.com/s3.everymomentcounts.com/wp-content/uploads/2020/12/17190530/3_PublicHealthApproach_11-07-20_AB_FINAL.pdf

Bazyk, S., Myers, S., Romaniw, A., Virone M., Greene, S., Fette, C., Thomas, L., Test, L., Thorman, J., & Rupp, T. (2022). ESSA OT Advocacy Network: Public health framework. Every Moment Counts. https://s3.us-east-2.amazonaws.com/s3.everymomentcounts.com/wp-content/uploads/2022/05/03202525/FINAL_OT_Role_ESSA_4-25-22_LONG.pdf

Bedell, G. M. (2012). Measurement of social participation. In V. Anderson & M. H. Beauchamp (Eds.), *Developmental social neuroscience and childhood brain insult: Theory and practice* (pp. 184-206). Guilford Press.

Cole, M., & Tufano, R. (2020). *Applied theories in occupational therapy: A practical approach* (2nd ed.). SLACK Incorporated.

Cook, G. (2013, October 22). *Why we are wired to connect*. Scientific American. https://www.scientificamerican.com/article/why-we-are-wired-to-connect/

De Las Heras, C. Geist, R. Kielhofner, G., & Yanling, L. (2007). *The Volitional Questionnaire*. The Model of Human Occupation Clearinghouse.

Donahue, M. (2013). *The social profile: Assessment of participation in children, adolescents, and adults*. AOTA Press.

Gable, S. L., & Haidt, J. (2005). What (and why) is positive psychology? *Review of General Psychology, 9(2)*, 103-110. https://doi.org/10.1037/1089-2680.9.2.103

Goleman, D. (1996). *Emotional intelligence: Why it can matter more than IQ*. Bloomsbury.

Goren, C., Satry, M., & Wu, P. (1975). Visual following and pattern discrimination and face-like stimuli by newborn infants. *Pediatrics, 56*(4), 544-549.

Hawkley, L., & Cacioppo, J. (2010). Loneliness matters: A theoretical and empirical review of consequences and mechanisms. *Annals of Behavioral Medicine, 40*(2), 218-227. https://doi.org/10.1007%2Fs12160-010-9210-8

Holt-Lunstad, J., Smith, T., & Layton, B. (2010). Social relationships and mortality risk: A meta-analysis. *PLOS Medicine, 7*(7), e1000316. https://doi.org/10.1371/journal.pmed.100316

Ikiugu, M. (2012). Use of theoretical conceptual practice models by occupational therapists the U.S.: A pilot study. *International Journal of Therapy and Rehabilitation, 11*, 629-639. https://doi.org/10.12968/ijtr.2012.19.11.629

Ikiugu, M., & Smallfield, S. (2015). Instructing occupational therapy students in use of theory to guide practice. *Occupational Therapy in Healthcare, 29*(2), 165-177. https://doi.org/10.3109/07380577.2015.1017787

Ikiugu, M., Smallfield, S., & Condit, C. (2009). A framework for combining theoretical conceptual practice models in occupational therapy practice. *Canadian Journal of Occupational Therapy, 76*(3), 162-170. https://doi.org/10.1177/000841740907600305

Khetani, M. A., & Coster, W. (2019). Social participation. In B. A. B. Schell & G. Gillen (Eds.), *Willard and Spackman's occupational therapy* (13th ed., pp. 847-860). Wolters Kluwer.

Koller, J. R., & Bertel, J. M. (2006). Responding to today's mental health needs of children, families and schools: Revisiting the preservice training and preparation of school-based personnel. *Education and Treatment of Children, 29*, 197-217.

Kronenberg, F., & Pollard, N. (2006). Political dimensions of occupation and the roles of occupational thera-py. *American Journal of Occupational Therapy, 60*(6), 617-625. https://doi.org/10.5014/ajot.60.6.617

Magasi, S., & Hammel, J. (2004). Social support and social network mobilization in African American women who have experienced strokes. *Disabilities Studies Quarterly, 24*(4). https://doi.org/10.18061/dsq.v24i4.878

Masia-Warner, C., Nangle, D. W., & Hansen, D. J. (2006). Bringing evidence-based child mental health services to the schools: General issues and specific populations. *Education and Treatment of Children, 29,* 165-172. https://doi.org/10.18061/dsq.v24i4.878

Mayer, J. D., Roberts, R. D., & Barasades, S. G. (2008). Human abilities: Emotional intelligence. *Annual Review of Psychology, 59,* 507-536. https://doi.org/10.1146/annurev.psych.59.103006.093646

Mayer, J. D., & Salovey, P. (2004). Social intelligence [emotional intelligence, personal intelligence]. In C. Peterson & M. E. P. Seligman (Eds.), *Character strengths and virtues* (pp. 337-353). American Psychological Association.

Mosey, A. C. (1986). *Psychological components of occupational therapy.* Raven Press.

O'Brien, J., & Kielhofner, G. (2017). The interaction between the person and the environment. In R. R. Taylor (Ed.), *Kielhofner's Model of Human Occupation* (5th ed., pp. 24-37). Wolters Kluwer Health.

Seligman, M. E. P. (2002). *Authentic happiness.* Free Press.

Seligman, M. E. P., & Csikszentmihalyi, M. (2000). Positive psychology: An introduction. *American Psychologist, 55,* 5-14. https://doi.org/10.1037/0003-066x.55.1.5

Taylor, R. (2017). *Kielhofner's Model of Human Occupation* (5th ed.). Wolters Kluwer.

World Health Organization. (2008). *International classification of functioning, disability and health.* Author.

12

Implementing and Advocating for a Theory-Based Practice

Francine M. Seruya, PhD, OTR/L, FAOTA
and Patricia Laverdure, OTD, OTR/L, BCP, FAOTA

Chapter Objectives

1. Understand the role mentorship plays in the application of theory into practice.
2. Describe models of practice that support collaborative and contextually based interventions.
3. Examine various models of service delivery for their utility in collaboration and moving theory into practice.

The use of theory as part of the professional reasoning, treatment planning, and intervention process is essential in developing an intentional practice with an emphasis on occupation. Using an occupation-based, organizing model in conjunction with complementary models addresses the need to have flexibility when making clinical decisions and allows practitioners to purposefully determine how the occupational strengths and challenges their students demonstrate can be best addressed to facilitate engagement and participation in their school day (Ikiugu & Smallfield, 2011). The format presented by this book demonstrates the practical application of many typically utilized models and frames of reference (FORs) used within occupational therapy as well as in school-based practice.

Although we have argued this model of professional reasoning and intervention provides a strong foundation to demonstrate the distinct value and efficacy of occupational therapy intervention, we acknowledge that many practitioners continue to need support implementing these recommendations because research has indicated a small percentage of practitioners readily incorporate

Laverdure, P., & Seruya, F. M. *Theory in School-Based Occupational Therapy Practice: A Practical Application* (pp. 165-174). DOI: 10.4324/9781003526773-12

theory into their decision making and practice (O'Neal et al., 2007) and that even when implementing theories within practice, practitioners are not easily able to explain the concepts and how the model effects change (Brown et al., 2009; Roger et al., 2005). Furthermore, the understanding of models and FORs has been construed as a means of explaining what we do to novice occupational therapy practitioners and potentially seen as something that does not hold value once someone has been practicing over time (Nash & Mitchell, 2017). Despite these perceptions, we suggest understanding and being able to implement theory-based models in practice is a means by which to strengthen professional identity as well as ensure interventions are occupation focused, especially when working within school-based settings (Towns & Ashby, 2014).

The model of theory selection and implementation suggested in this book acknowledges that practitioners feel that there is no single model or frame that adequately addresses the needs of their clients (Green, 2000). Furthermore, the application of multiple models needs to be done in an intentional and well-thought-out manner rather than via "eclectic" practice (Ikiugu, 2012) or by relying on technical skills (Forsyth & Hamilton, 2005). Therefore, we argue that the act of providing knowledge via traditional teaching in didactic, entry-level occupational therapy education is not adequate in and of itself to ensure that knowledge is applied in intervention. Further reinforcement of these concepts via mentorship is needed to allow new practitioners the opportunity for modeling and guidance when applying theories to the school setting. In addition to mentorship and having the ability to model the use of theory as a guide to practice, exploring different service delivery models that are more complementary to collaborative and contextually based practice also supports the use of theories when reasoning evaluation and interventions.

This chapter intends to aid practitioners in making these decision-making models part of their daily practice as well as working to advocate for the use of theory-based practice within their settings. Additionally, the authors tie in how professionalism, knowledge translation, and the use of theory are intertwined and the importance of using mentors and social learning to facilitate the use of theory into practice and bolster professionalism and professional identity for practitioners. Finally, a discussion of collaborative, contextual-based practices within the school setting as a means of creating relationships with other professionals to promote shared understanding is also provided.

DEVELOPING PROFESSIONAL IDENTITY THROUGH KNOWLEDGE TRANSLATION AND MENTORSHIP

Knowledge translation is the process by which research is created and generated and then flows to implementation (Sudsawad, 2007). The term was first coined by the Canadian Institutes of Health Research in 2000 whereby the definition of knowledge translation was articulated as "the exchange, synthesis and ethically-sound application of knowledge—within a complex system of interactions among researchers and users—to accelerate the capture of the benefits of research for Canadians through improved health, more effective services and products, and a strengthened health care system" (Canadian Institutes of Health Research, 2005, para. 2). Since its introduction, knowledge translation has been adopted by many national and global health organizations such as the World Health Organization (Sudsawad, 2007). Regardless of the agency, the concepts have remained generally the same with the focus on how knowledge, typically generated via traditional research methods, is then implemented into everyday practice within health care systems as a means of bridging the evidence to practice gap.

Knowledge translation has been embraced in the field of occupational therapy as one that allows for more inclusive types of research, such as qualitative research, and addresses the systemic nature in which much of the occupational therapy research is conducted (Clark et al., 2013). Therefore, the use of a knowledge translation paradigm is more inclusive of the more typical types of research conducted within occupational therapy and also allows for the use of other forms of evidence such as that of the more rigorous research notions as posited when looking at evidence-based practice guidelines (Lencucha et al., 2007). In addition to knowledge translation as a means by which to bridge the evidence to practice gap, implementation science has also been viewed as a vehicle by which we can facilitate the use of research findings and other evidence-based practices into routine clinical practice to improve the quality and effectiveness of services (Eccles & Mittman, 2006). Therefore, implementation science is viewed as another viable model of knowledge translation for moving research into practice in a timely and efficient manner.

Model of Knowledge Translation

Models of knowledge translation include 4 main stages: (a) planning/design (identifies a knowledge gap, engages stakeholders, and develops an intervention), (b) implementation, (c) evaluation, and (d) sustainability (Eccles & Mittman, 2006). We can use these stages to effectively address how we can move theory more readily into practice. Engaging students and colleagues in discussions related to clinical reasoning and framing the strength and challenges of the child or children in terms of an occupation-based model can begin the process of problem identification, engagement, and development of intervention. Through collaboration, occupational therapy practitioners and teachers can identify existing challenges and begin to determine the overarching, organizing model of practice to address the identified issues. Using the organizing model, further identification of complementary models can be highlighted to address more specific challenges or barriers to participation. Implementing the intervention based on the assumptions and postulates of the organizing and complementary models can occur with the ability to predict changes. Evaluation of the alignment of the assumptions of the model with treatment and goal attainment to determine efficacy of the intervention in eliciting the desired outcomes will guide future interventions. Finally, occupational therapy practitioners can continually use this method as a sustained means by which they can implement intentional clinical reasoning to make further refinement or subsequent changes in order to meet the needs of the child or population within the school. The use of knowledge translation and implementation science offers possible ways of framing the means by which occupational therapy practitioners can collaborate with teachers to bridge the theory to practice gap while implementing models and frames within their practice. Another factor to consider when translating professional knowledge is the role of mentorship in developing the next generation of practitioners.

DEVELOPING THE NEXT GENERATION OF THEORY-BASED OCCUPATIONAL THERAPY PRACTITIONERS

Research has demonstrated that students are highly influenced by their clinical preceptors. Clinical placements provide an opportunity for students to engage in real-time clinical reasoning while under the direct supervision of a mentor. The American Occupational Therapy Association (AOTA) requires a minimum of 1 year of experience for an individual to take on supervision and mentorship of a student from an educational program (Accreditation Council for Occupational Therapy Education, 2018). The internship or fieldwork process capitalizes on the assumptions of social learning theory whereby students learn by modeling the behaviors they observe in their supervisors. Not only does this apply to technical skills such as activity analysis, goal writing, and activity selection but also to the use of theory. Students who have clinical preceptors who are able to articulate and engage their students in dialogue about the use of theory-guided practice leads to students who are more comfortable in understanding how to implement these models within their clinical practice and understand the clinical utility of using such theories (Nash & Mitchell, 2017). Likewise, when clinical preceptors do not emphasize the use of theory in practice, students often voice dissatisfaction related to the time spent in their educational programs on theory (Hodgetts et al., 2007). Therefore, evidence suggests that clinical fieldwork supervisors as well as clinical mentors have a vital role in continuing the development of intentional occupational therapy practitioners who ground themselves in theory when engaging in the occupational therapy process. This is an important consideration, as we have posited throughout this text, because the use of theory not only provides the basis for the occupational therapy process, but it also provides the underpinnings for professional identity.

EMBRACING OUR PROFESSIONAL IDENTITY

Improving professional identity as well as professional recognition is an important facet of school-based practice. As previously noted, the role of school-based occupational therapy practitioners is frequently misunderstood, and their scope of practice is often underestimated, with interventions related to the development of handwriting or sensory processing being the most notably linked with occupational therapy practitioners (Seruya & Garfinkel, 2020). The ability to use models and FORs to demonstrate the robust theoretical foundations of interventions not only provides increased credence to the occupational therapy process but also illuminates the distinct value occupational therapy brings to the educational team. Additionally, articulating foundations to practice as well as the distinct contribution of occupational therapy can help to bolster the individual occupational therapy practitioner's professional identity and the continued development of professionalism within in the clinical setting.

The teaching and development of professionalism and professional values begin in didactic education and are reinforced through clinical education. Although professionalism is highly regarded and considered an essential skill, the nuances of professionalism can be difficult to teach. Acknowledging the difficulty of teaching professionalism to entry-level students, Chien and colleagues (2020) used a method in which they tied theory development to professional development by having students reach out to interview practitioners in the field who had contributed to the development of a model or theory within the profession. Their results indicated that, by interacting with this individual, students' conceptions of what it means to be a professional as well as their overall reflection of their own professionalism grew. In this example, attaching theory to the concepts of professionalism helped to bolster the understanding of how the concepts support each other. Using theory as a vehicle to tie professionalism and professional values to practice allows occupational therapy practitioners the continued opportunity to educate and advocate for the profession.

COLLABORATION AND SHARED DECISION MAKING

As part of best practice, practitioners are encouraged to engage in collaborative partnerships with the other professionals who are part of the school team (AOTA, 2017). The provision of services in collaboration with other team members offers extensive opportunities for occupational therapy practitioners to articulate and demonstrate their scope of practice. Working collaboratively also offers occupational therapy practitioners a means by which they can articulate how occupation-based theories and FORs support the clinical-reasoning processes used for decision making in evaluation and treatment. The literature in occupational therapy is extensive in relation to the need for and the exploration of collaborative practices.

In many cases, collaboration in the school setting has been largely viewed from the perspective of the occupational therapy practitioner collaborating with classroom teachers as well as other teachers such as those from physical education and art. Collaboration in school settings has been a somewhat enigmatic endeavor and was initially carried out more in a consultative manner rather than a collaborative one (Bose & Hinojosa, 2008; Rose & Seruya, 2020). Occupational therapy practitioners providing biomechanical or neurologic rationales for recommendations and subsequent adaptive tools such as pencil grips and slant boards were often the extent of the collaboration between the occupational therapy practitioner and the teacher. This model of intervention places the occupational therapy practitioner in more of an "expert" role, providing to the teacher the knowledge or assistive technology they believe will address barriers or challenges the child may be having. Although this type of information and equipment can be deemed important to the therapeutic intervention and aid children in accessing their curriculum, the manner in which these are provided is essential to consider. Developing collaborative relationships with classroom teachers and other school personnel is an essential component to effective intervention (Frolek Clark & Polichino, 2021; Seruya & Garfinkel, 2020). Despite the evidence supporting the use of collaborative and contextually based intervention, nonintegrated models continue to prevail when assessing typical practice patterns of school-based occupational therapy practitioners (Seruya & Garfinkel, 2020). The use of nonintegrated (or "pull out") models of intervention support this type of interaction because time is limited when needing to take children to and from classrooms.

Contextual-Based Services

Current practices emphasize the importance of contextually based (or "push in") services because they are aligned with best practices (AOTA, 2017) and support the tenets of providing services in the least restrictive environment as mandated by the Individuals with Disabilities Education Act (2004). As the shift to more integrated service delivery models has become more prevalent (Seruya & Garfinkel, 2020), the need to improve occupational therapy practitioners' aptitude in developing collaborative intervention approaches has increased (Friedman et al., 2022; Laverdure et al., 2016; Seruya & Garfnkel, 2018). Occupational therapy practitioners often face a variety of challenges and barriers when attempting to implement collaborative and contextually based practices.

Practitioners cite a lack of time, poor administrative support, and high caseloads as typical barriers to adapting current practice patterns (Seruya & Garfinkel, 2020). A lack of role clarity also affects the ability of occupational therapy practitioners to perform within the range of their scope of practice (Artale-Morgante & Seruya, 2017; Lamash & Fogel, 2021). Although there is literature exploring the practices of collaboration within schools between occupational therapy practitioners and teachers and supporting the need for contextually based inclusive practices, there are few guidelines available or evidence supporting the positive outcomes related to collaboration between occupational therapy practitioners and classroom teachers.

Contextually Based and Integrated Service Model

To provide a pragmatic and directive approach to collaboration, Seruya and Garfinkel (2018) proposed a model of contextually based service delivery that is based not on the occupational therapy practitioner as the expert but rather on the occupational therapy practitioner and the teacher as equals and that is based on the open system theory for their Contextually Based and Integrated Service model (Figure 12-1). Using this model, occupational therapy practitioners and teachers work together to identify barriers and challenges, explore the environment in which the challenges occur, provide contextually based intervention based on mutual problem solving, and then use feedback to assess the outcome and begin the process over. Their model outlines three specific action steps to guide the occupational therapy practitioner's and teacher's interactions: (a) information exchange, (b) analysis of context, and (c) problem solving and planning. Each step is further elaborated on through the use of feedback. Using this model, an occupational therapy practitioner, as part of information exchange, may begin to formulate theoretical suppositions based on information received from the teacher related to occupational strengths and challenges. The occupational therapy practitioner can reason out the alignment of these assumptions through dialogue with the teacher to reach consensus regarding appropriate theoretical foundations. As they move into exploration of context, occupational therapy practitioners can share clinical reasoning related to more targeted models and FORs that support participation in the various contexts in which participation is expected. As interventions are implemented within the contextual setting, occupational therapy practitioners and teachers have the opportunity to problem solve and plan interventions within the context of the classroom, basing those interventions on sound theoretical foundations. Because the teacher has been a part of the planning and the clinical, theoretical reasoning to develop the intervention, there is increased opportunity for them to gain further insight into the larger scope of practice and increase their level of knowledge and understanding of the occupational therapy process. Throughout the process, the occupational therapy practitioner and teacher work to provide feedback to each other and on the proposed interventions to provide the best outcomes for students. This model provides ample opportunity for occupational therapy practitioners to use models and theories as a way to plan intervention as well as provide education about and advocate for the distinct value of the profession.

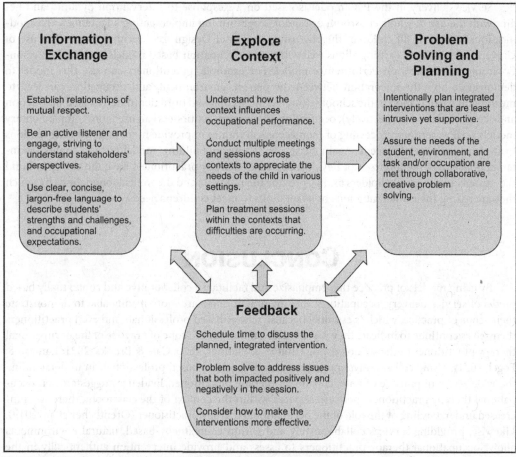

Figure 12-1. The Contextually Based and Integrated Service model. (Reproduced with permission from Seruya, F. M., & Garfinkel, M. [2018]. Implementing contextually based services: Where do we begin? *SIS Quarterly Practice Connections,* 3[3], 4-6.)

Partnering for Change Model

In a more population-based approach, Missiuna and colleagues (2012) developed a contextually based model that supported capacity building to address service provision to children with special needs via collaboration and coaching. Partnering For Change (P4C; Missiuna et al., 2012), similar to the Contextually Based and Integrated Service model, promotes active problem solving between the teacher and the occupational therapy practitioner and supports the provision of services within the context of the classroom. The foundation of the model lies in the concepts of relationship building and knowledge translation. For example, the development of collaborative relationships between occupational therapy practitioners, teachers, parents, and students is enabled through the use of education sessions regarding the scope of practice and the role of occupational therapy practitioners based on the identified needs of the student or teacher. Occupational therapy practitioners can use these sessions to explain various theories and models of practice to demonstrate how they address barriers to participation. By using strategies aligned with knowledge translation, the occupational therapy practitioner can facilitate problem solving and implementing strategies within the context of the classroom. The occupational therapy practitioner can provide the theoretical basis for the selection of various intervention strategies and have the opportunity to not only explain but also model the use of the theory in developing active classroom strategies and interventions.

Service delivery in the P4C model is based on a Response to Intervention pyramid and begins with the use of whole classroom or school programming implementing adaptations and modifications benefiting all children, thereby using Universal Design for Learning tenets. The use of Universal Design for Learning aligns well with many occupation-based models such as the Person-Environment-Occupation-Performance model. For example, practitioners can use this model to demonstrate how the integration between the person, environment, and occupation can lead to meaningful participation in the school setting. At the second and third tier (differentiated instruction and accommodation, respectively), occupational therapy practitioners can use more complementary models such as sensory processing or biomechanical frames to provide more targeted interventions to students with specific needs. Again, because relationship building, modeling, and contextual interventions are at the forefront of P4C, occupational therapy practitioners have the ability to build the capacity of other stakeholders as they provide the rationale and theoretical foundations by which they are basing their differentiations or adaptations to meet children's needs.

CONCLUSION

By using models of practice that emphasize and facilitate a collaborative and contextually based model of service delivery, occupational therapy practitioners are more readily able to demonstrate their scope of practice, which is essential because school-based professionals and even practitioners themselves continue to indicate they are not clear on the role or scope of practice of the occupational therapy practitioner in the school setting (Bolton & Plattner, 2020; Caie & Brooks, 2021; Lamash & Fogel, 2021). Using collaborative models assists other school-based professionals in understanding the wide scope of practice of an occupational therapy practitioner. Evidence suggests when occupational therapy practitioners perform services within the context of the classroom, there is an increased understanding of the role of the occupational therapy practitioner (Orentlicher et al., 2019). Likewise, providing services collaboratively and within contextually based, natural environments allows occupational therapy practitioners to assess and provide intervention authentically in the setting in which students are expected to perform. This type of collaboration facilitates the ability to conduct occupation-based and client-centered assessment and intervention.

REFERENCES

Accreditation Council for Occupational Therapy Education. (2018). 2018 ACOTE Standards and interpretive guide. https://acoteonline.org/accreditation-explained/standards/

American Occupational Therapy Association. (2017). Guidelines for occupational therapy services in early intervention and schools. *American Journal of Occupational Therapy, 71*(Suppl. 2), 7112410010p1-7112410010p10. https://doi.org/10.5014/ajot.2017.716S01

Artale-Morgante, M., & Seruya, F. M. (2017). Developing inclusive school communities: An expanded role for school-based occupational therapy. *American Journal of Occupational Therapy, 71*(4 Suppl. 1), 7111515230pl-7111515230pl. https://doi.org/10.5014/ajot.2017.71S1-PO3091

Bolton, T., & Plattner, L. (2020). Occupational therapy role in school-based practice: Perspectives from teachers and OTs. *Journal of Occupational Therapy, Schools, & Early Intervention, 13*(2), 136-146. https://doi.org/10.1080/19411243.2019.1636749

Bose, P., & Hinojosa, J. (2008). Reported experiences from occupational therapists interacting with teachers in inclusive early childhood classrooms. *American Journal of Occupational Therapy, 62*(3), 289-297. https://doi.org/10.5014/ajot.62.3.289

Brown, T., Rodger, S., Brown, A., & Roever, C. (2009). A profile of Canadian pediatric occupational therapy practice. *Occupational Therapy in Health Care, 21*(4), 39-69. https://doi.org/10.1080/J003v21n04_03

Canadian Institutes of Health Research (2005). About knowledge translation. http://www.cihr-irsc.gc.ca/e/29418. html

Caie, P., & Brooks, R. (2021). We need to completely change the way we look at therapy: Occupational therapy in specialist schools. *Journal of Occupational Therapy, Schools & Early Intervention, 15*(4), 1-13.

Chien, C.-W., Chloe Mo, S. Y., & Chow, J. (2020). Using an international role-modeling pedagogy to engage first-year occupational therapy students in learning professionalism. *American Journal of Occupational Therapy, 74*, 7406205060. https://doi.org/10.5014/ajot.2020.039859

Clark, F., Park, D. J., & Burke, J. P. (2013). Dissemination: Bringing translational research to completion. *American Journal of Occupational Therapy, 67*, 185-193. https://doi.org/10.5014/ajot.2013.006148

Eccles, M. P., & Mittman, B. S. (2006). Welcome to implementation science. *Implementation Science, 1*, 1. https://doi.org/10.1186/1748-5908-1-1

Forsyth, K., & Hamilton, E. (2005). Social service occupational therapists' view of practice and integration with health: A survey. *British Journal of Occupational Therapy, 71*(2), 64-71.

Friedman, Z. L., Hubbard, H., & Seruya, F. M. (2022). Building better teams: Impact of education and coaching intervention on interprofessional collaboration between teachers and occupational therapists in schools. *Journal of Occupational Therapy, Schools, & Early Intervention, 16*(2), 173-193. https://doi.org/10.1080/19411243.2022.2037492

Frolek Clark, G., & Polichino, J. (2021). School occupational therapy: Staying focused on participation and educational performance. *Journal of Occupational Therapy, Schools, & Early Intervention, 14*(1), 19-26.

Green, J. (2000). The role of theory in evidence-based health promotion practice. *Health Education Research, 15*(2), 125-129.

Hodgetts, S., Hollis, V., Triska, O., Dennis, S., Madill, H., & Taylor, E. (2007). Occupational therapy students' and graduates' satisfaction with professional education and preparedness for practice. *Canadian Journal of Occupational Therapy, 74*, 148-160. https://doi.org/10.1177/000841740707400303

Ikiugu, M. (2012). Use of theoretical conceptual practice models by occupational therapists in the US: A pilot study. *International Journal of Therapy and Rehabilitation, 19*(11), 629-637. https://doi.org/10.12968/ijtr.2012.19.11.629

Ikiugu, M., & Smallfield, S. (2011). Ikiugu's eclectic method of combining theoretical conceptual practice models in occupational therapy. *Australian Occupational Therapy Journal, 58*(6), 437-446. https://doi.org/10.1111/j.1440-1630.2011.00968.x

Individuals with Disabilities Education Act of 2004, Pub. L. 108-446, 20 U.S.C. §1400 et seq (2004).

Lamash, L., & Fogel, Y. (2021). Role perception and professional identity of occupational therapists working in education systems. *Canadian Journal of Occupational Therapy, 88*(2), 163-172.

Laverdure, P., Seruya, F. M., Stephenson, P., & Cosbey, J. (2016). Paradigm transitions in pediatric practice: Tools to guide practice. *SIS Quarterly Practice Connections, 1*(2), 5-7.

Lencucha, R., Kothari, A., & Rouse, M. (2007). The issue is—Knowledge translation: A concept for occupational therapy? *American Journal of Occupational Therapy, 61*, 593-596.

Missiuna, C. A., Pollock, N. A., Levac, D. E., Campbell, W. N., Whalen, S. D., Bennett, S. M., Hecimovich, C. A., Gaines, B. R., Cairney, J., & Russell, D. J. (2012). Partnering for change: An innovative school-based occupational therapy service delivery model for children with developmental coordination disorder. *Canadian Journal of Occupational Therapy, 79*, 41-50. https://doi.org/10.2182/cjot.2012.79.1.6

Nash, B. H., & Mitchell, A. W. (2017). Longitudinal study of changes in occupational therapy students' perspectives on frames of reference. *American Journal of Occupational Therapy, 71*, 7105230010. https://doi.org/10.5014/ ajot.2017.024455

O'Neal, S., Dickerson, A. E., & Holbert, D. (2007). The use of theory by occupational therapists working with adults with developmental disabilities. *Occupational Therapy in Health Care, 21*(4), 71-85. https://doi.org/10.1080/J003v21n04_04

Orentlicher, M., Lashinsky, D., Teixeira, S. B., & Mograby, A. (2019). The experiences and perceptions of collaboration between OTs and other school professionals. *American Journal of Occupational Therapy, 73*(4 Suppl. ll), 7311505127p1-7311505127p1. https://doi.org/10.5014/ ajot.2019.73SI-PO4003

Roger, S., Brown, T., & Brown, A. (2005). Profile of paediatric occupational therapy practice in Australia. *Australian Occupational Therapy Journal, 52*, 311-325.

Rose, E., & Seruya, F. M. (2020). Collaboration, the elusive phenomenon: Perceptions of OTs in the school setting. *American Journal of Occupational Therapy, 74*(4 Suppl. 1), 747411505134. https://doi.org/10.5014/ ajot.2020.74S1-PO3315

Seruya, F. M., & Garfinkel, M. (2018). Implementing contextually based services: Where do we begin? *SIS Quarterly Practice Connections, 3*(3), 4-6.

Seruya, F. M., & Garfinkel, M. (2020). Caseload and workload: Current trends in school-based practice across the United States. *American Journal of Occupational Therapy, 74*(5), 1-8. https://doi.org/10.5014/ajot.2020.039818

Sudsawad, P. (2007). *Knowledge translation: Introduction to models, strategies, and measures.* Southwest Educational Development Laboratory, National Center for the Dissemination of Disability Research.

Towns, E., & Ashby, S. (2014). The influence of practice educators on occupational therapy students' understanding of the practical applications of theoretical knowledge: A phenomenological study into student experiences of practice education. *Australian Occupational Therapy Journal, 61*(5), 344-352. https://doi.org/10.1111/1440-1630.12134

FINANCIAL DISCLOSURES

Dr. Tammy Blake reported no financial or proprietary interest in the materials presented herein.

Dr. Mindy Garfinkel reported no financial or proprietary interest in the materials presented herein.

Dr. Moses N. Ikiugu reported no financial or proprietary interest in the materials presented herein.

Dr. Paula Kramer reported no financial or proprietary interest in the materials presented herein.

Dr. Patricia Laverdure reported no financial or proprietary interest in the materials presented herein.

Dr. Deborah Schwind reported no financial or proprietary interest in the materials presented herein.

Dr. Francine M. Seruya reported no financial or proprietary interest in the materials presented herein.

Dr. Caitlin Stanford reported no financial or proprietary interest in the materials presented herein.

Dr. Miranda Virone reported no financial or proprietary interest in the materials presented herein.

Dr. Tina Weisman reported no financial or proprietary interest in the materials presented herein.

INDEX

Printed in the United States
by Baker & Taylor Publisher Services

Printed in the United States
by Baker & Taylor Publisher Services